Psychosocial Aspects of End-Stage Renal Disease: Issues of Our Times

Psychosocial Aspects of End-Stage Renal Disease: Issues of Our Times

Mark A. Hardy, John Kiernan,
Austin H. Kutscher, Lynn Cahill,
and Alan I. Benvenisty
Editors

With the editorial assistance of
Jill C. Crabtree

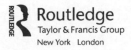

Routledge
Taylor & Francis Group
New York   London

Psychosocial Aspects of End-Stage Renal Disease: Issues of Our Times has also been published as *Loss, Grief & Care,* Volume 5, Numbers 1/2 1991.

The Haworth Press, Inc., 10 Alice Street, Binghamton, NY 13904-1580
EUROSPAN/Haworth, 3 Henrietta Street, London WC2E 8LU England
ASTAM/Haworth, 162-168 Parramatta Road, Stanmore, Sydney, N.S.W. 2048 Australia

This edition by Routledge:

Routledge
Taylor and Francis Group
270 Madison Avenue
New York, NY 10016

Routledge
Taylor and Francis Group
2 Park Square, Milton Park
Abingdon, Oxon OX14 4RN

Library of Congress Cataloging-in-Publication Data

Psychosocial aspects of end-stage renal disease: issues of our times/Mark A. Hardy . . .[et al.], editors; with editorial assistance of Jill C. Crabtree.
    p. cm.
    "Has also been published as Loss, grief & care, volume 5, numbers 1/2, 1991" — T.p. verso.
    ISBN 1-56024-149-7 (alk. paper)
    1. Chronic renal failure — Social aspects. 2. Chronic renal failure — Psychological aspects. 3. Chronic renal failure — Treatment — Moral and ethical aspects. I. Hardy, Mark A. (Mark Adam), 1938- .
    [DNLM: 1. Ethics, Medical. 2. Hemodialysis — psychology. 3. Kidney Failure, Acute — psychology. 4. Kidney Failure, Acute — therapy. 5. Kidney Failure, Chronic — psychology. 6. Kidney Failure, Chronic — therapy. 7. Quality of Life. 8. Social Support. W1 LO853F v. 5 no. 1/ 2 / WJ 342 P9745]
RC918.R4P79 1991
616.6'14 — dc20
DNLM/DLC
for Library of Congress
                                    91-7041
                                         CIP

Psychosocial Aspects
of End-Stage Renal Disease:
Issues of Our Times

CONTENTS

IV. STAFF/PATIENT PERSPECTIVES IN CARE OF RENAL DISEASE

V. RENAL DISEASE AND SPECIAL PATIENT POPULATIONS

ABOUT THE EDITORS

Mark A. Hardy, MD, Professor of Surgery, College of Physicians and Surgeons, Columbia University, New York, New York.

John Kiernan, MBA, (Health Administration), former Administrator and Coordinator, Organ Recovery Program, The Presbyterian Hospital in the City of New York; Regulatory Affairs Analyst, ICD-International Center for the Disabled, New York, New York.

Austin H. Kutscher, PhD, President, The Foundation of Thanatology, New York, New York; Professor of Dentistry (in Psychiatry), Department of Psychiatry, College of Physicians and Surgeons, School of Dental and Oral Surgery, Columbia University, New York, New York.

Lynn Cahill, MSW, Department of Social Work Services, Presbyterian Hospital in the City of New York, New York, New York.

Alan I. Benvenisty, MD, Assistant Professor of Surgery, College of Physicians and Surgeons, Columbia University, New York, New York.

The publication of this book was supported in part by a grant from the Lucius N. Littauer Foundation.

INTRODUCTION

Communication Between the Disciplines in Care of Patients with End-Stage Renal Disease

Austin H. Kutscher

Over 21 years ago, The Foundation of Thanatology was organized to build a very special kind of bridge—a communications bridge in the practice area of thanatology—for professionals in the allied health services and for those who came to them for help. Although bridges are usually constructed to create linkages between different geographic locations and different individuals, it was evident that this communications bridge would have to be built, not with bricks and mortar, but with ideas and words. Notwithstanding the tremendous advances made in medical technology in multiple diseases, communication between the disciplines in the allied health sciences, and between the members of these disciplines and patients, was grossly deficient. As the capacity of science to prolong

Austin H. Kutscher is President of the Foundation of Thanatology and is Professor of Dentistry (in Psychiatry), Department of Psychiatry, College of Physicians and Surgeons, Columbia University, New York, NY.

1

life for those who were life-threatened expanded, the indignities imposed upon both patients and their family members increased. Technology seemed to promise a cure for all diseases, but in the pursuit of this promise, too often the humanitarian dimensions of patient caregiving were overwhelmed by the protocols of biophysiological science.

The first problems communicated in the effort to treat the whole patient and not just the disease were those of the cancer patient. You are all familiar with the paradigm of the "five stages" that at one point seemed to describe all patients in the course of a life-threatening and ultimately fatal illness. Whether or not we can accept the Kübler-Ross design for all disease states and all trajectories of dying, we can acknowledge that its importance is its stress on the personhood of the patient and not on the symptomatology of the disease.

In its own attempt to pursue this same course and to arrive at some degree of resolution, The Foundation of Thanatology embarked on a program of symposia and publications that communicated not only the dilemmas of the world of cancer but also those that became apparent in other long-term and chronic disorders among a broad range of patients, including children as well as the elderly.

We have come now to end-stage renal disease, where, certainly, technology is giving much hope for quality in living, where caregivers are expressing great concern for maintaining this quality of life, and where legislation on the national level is fulfilling a financial commitment to those suffering from this chronic and long-term illness. What has been achieved should serve as a model approach, if not the definitive one, for other illnesses.

The communications bridge that we will traverse in this publication will, we hope, enable many disciplines not only to share their knowledge but also to reveal the problems that are still evident to them in the confrontation with potentially fatal illness. In planning this volume, we have enlisted the collaboration of interdisciplinary leaders. It could be said that they are true pioneers, since during their professional lives, almost miraculous events have come to pass: the successful transplantation of organs; the introduction of drugs that reduce the incidence of organ rejection; better technologies in dialysis to sustain those unable for any reason to benefit from a transplanted kidney; an organization for the procuring of these organs; and involvement of researchers, clinicians, and staff in the unending challenge to improve the quality of the lives they are saving.

I. RENAL DISEASE AND THE FAMILY

End-Stage Renal Disease: Family Responses

Katherine M. Steckler
Florence E. Selder

End-stage renal disease (ESRD) takes a significant toll on the patient and the family. However, more is known about the multiple affronts the disease has for the patient than about the disease's impact on the family unit.

The role of the family in the course of recurrent and chronic illness has been examined within two views. One approach has focused on major crises and catastrophes in family life. A second approach focuses on the more subtle and persistent patterns of family interaction and process. A combination of these approaches was used in this study. The diagnosis of the disease was treated as the initial point, and the ensuing family interaction and process was the focus of the study.

A pilot study was conducted to gather patient and family responses. Selection criteria for the patient subjects were that all sub-

Katherine M. Steckler, RN, MS, is affiliated with the Milwaukee County Mental Health Complex, Milwaukee, WI. Florence E. Selder, RN, PhD, is Assistant Professor and Urban Research Center Scientist, University of Wisconsin, Milwaukee, WI.

jects be married and have at least one adult child. All patient subjects had undergone hemodialysis treatment for at least six months and had no other life-threatening illness in an exacerbated state. The criteria for the family member subjects were that the spouse be currently married to the patient and the adult child be at least 18 years of age. The total sample contained nine subjects. All subjects were Caucasian, with ages ranging from 22 to 64. The three patient subjects receiving hemodialysis treatments were the fathers of the three families. There were two adult male children and one female. Only the female adult child lived at home. None of the hemodialysis subjects was employed. One of the three spouses was employed. All of the children were employed. All patient subjects had some type of health care insurance. The length of the patient subjects' illnesses ranged from one year to eight years. The length of time the patient subjects had been receiving dialysis was from one year to six-and-a-half years. Data were collected through intensive interviewing and were analyzed using life transition theory.

The life transition theory was used to provide insights previously lacking in ESRD literature. For example, a frequent criticism of the reported literature on ESRD and the marital dyad and family responses is the absence of an interpersonal framework. The life transition theory provides for a description of individuals' responses and the interpersonal interactions of the dyad. Furthermore, the frameworks in the literature only account for the patient responses from a strictly psychological perspective. The language of life transition theory minimizes a strictly psychological interpretation of experiences.

Succinctly stated, the life transition is a passage that follows a reality that has been disrupted. The transition is a bridge from an existing reality to one of several possible realities. The task for the family unit in this transition is to integrate the ESRD and the treatment of dialysis in such a way that it has some meaning for them. The reality that will be ultimately structured will follow the previously held expectations. Throughout the transition there is also a regaining of one's sense of self. For individuals this sense of one's self is described as identity constancy, e.g., the stable state of being one's self. For the family members this is termed the family unit's identity, e.g., the stable state of being the family.

The major characteristic of a life transition is uncertainty. All subjects reported experiencing uncertainty during the time the diagnosis of end-stage renal disease was being made. For two of the families, the diagnosis and subsequent need for hemodialysis was not established at the onset of the illness. As one daughter said, "We didn't know what was wrong with him right away, but he didn't come home from the hospital for nine months . . . by the time . . . we realized he was to be on dialysis the rest of his life . . . it was like nothing compared to what we had just been through." A son said: ". . . they told us time and time again that he wasn't going to make it . . . on and on . . . it was almost a blessing that it finally came down."

Thus, the uncertainty was more pronounced in the process of being diagnosed than in the diagnosis itself. The families' differing perspectives also added to uncertainty. For instance, one patient subject reported, "I didn't feel close to anybody. I was fighting my own private war. I was just on my own." Whereas, his daughter reported, "Well, he just, well, it's like he won't do anything. He just walks around the house and makes a mess, and I think he's just trying to make more work for me . . . It's hard because I don't quite fully understand what he is feeling."

The ambiguity that accompanies a chronic illness and its continuous changes create further uncertainty. This was illustrated in a son's report of his father's changing condition. He said,

> . . . sometimes his changes are worse and sometimes better. He just keeps getting sick. Sometimes I don't think he's going to last a year, you know. Other times he really feels pretty good . . . . And six months ago, if you would have asked me, I wouldn't have figured he would have made it three months.

One of the children described the uncertainty incurred by an acute episode of the father's ESRD:

. . . between my mother, my brother, sister and myself going to the hospital every night, it was all so trying. It was like we were all so exhausted, we didn't know what to do. Every two or three nights the hospital would call. Everyone did not know what to do. We didn't know what to do . . .

In addition to the ongoing changes and acute upsets, the treatment options may also be a source of uncertainty. In selected cases, renal transplant may be offered to patients. This then creates a resurgence of uncertainty. As one patient said, "I don't want anything to do with a transplant or home dialysis. I consider this (hemodialysis) a sure thing and it's working. The uncertainty of a transplant is just too much."

Living with a family member on dialysis creates uncertainty in daily living. One wife said, "I don't plan ahead anymore. I don't know . . . what he's gonna feel like. I just can't make plans that far ahead."

In summary, uncertainty was reported by all subjects in this study. The sources of uncertainty were related to personal factors and to factors associated with the nature of the disease and its treatment.

According to life transition theory, once uncertainty is experienced, a number of processes will be undertaken to decrease it. First, information will be sought; initially, information decreases uncertainty. In this study subjects sought information from health care providers and available literature about the disease. People reported reading pamphlets from the Kidney Foundation and from the Veterans Administration Center. One son said; "Getting information from my mother and going over it was very helpful."

Another child said, "It's not like some story you read about, some tragic happening in a magazine. It's your life . . . I asked all kinds of questions. Doctors, nurses, I asked everybody. I didn't know anything . . . I had to ask to get the information."

Other comments included:

"We read the Kidney Foundation newsletter all the time."

"VA gave us a lot of little things, pamphlets and everything that they give you . . . you read."

"The most helpful thing was the willingness of the staff . . . to explain everything to us . . ."

Thus, all subjects initially sought information to reduce uncertainty. Once the uncertainty was reduced, people then attempted to come to terms with the permanency of the diagnosis, the treatment requirements, and the irreversibility of the disease.

To engage in a meaningful transition, persons must come to terms with the permanency and irreversibility of the disease through acknowledgment of its existence. Conditional acknowledgment is the admission of a fact, attenuated by a modifying circumstance; this enables a person to acknowledge that event while maintaining some qualifications. For example, a patient and/or members of the family may say, "There's always a miracle." In contrast, nonacknowledgment is the failure to acknowledge the event, the consequences of the event, or the changed circumstances brought on by the event. An example would be a man who is noncompliant in his treatment because he denies that he has ESRD. It is essential that the person acknowledge the irreversibility of the disease and begin to relinquish the previous reality of being disease-free. Refusing to acknowledge the permanency of the changed reality results in a failure to structure a new reality. Living as if one is not dependent on dialysis or does not have to comply with a treatment regime will compromise the one's health. In life transition theory, realizing the irreversibility of the disease and the changed reality is labeled irrevocability. Irrevocability coupled with reactivation are the two trigger events that precipitate an awareness of the dysfunctional reality and bring about recognition of the implication of change.

One subject commented on the irrevocability of the disease: "I didn't realize I'd be on it (hemodialysis) so long. I thought maybe three times. I'd be all right. But after the third time, I realized, it won't go away. Never. I thought it would—but it won't."

Another way of learning about the irreversibility of the disease is to identify what is no longer available to the person. These are called missed options. One patient subject reported, ". . . Well, I had a business . . . at one time I was the purchasing manager at the business . . . it was a rather active life, really. I might spend 12 to 14 hours a day at that place and having dropped off all of a sudden, I still miss it."

Several subjects reported missed options in terms of their family members or their own activities. A spouse reported, "He was always so active, active in athletics and of course, he's cut that out now."

In relation to social activities a spouse said, ". . . Well, I don't think we get out as much anymore with our friends because it's different . . . I find it a little bit difficult at times."

A second spouse reported a similar experience: ". . . Well, we were involved in a lot a things. We were busy. We kept busy with our kids and we were involved in church affairs. Then we cut back on all of that because he just wasn't up to it anymore."

One son said, "It's hard for them. Can't drink. Can't dance. If they go, they don't stay long. It's just not the same for them as far as their social life."

Missed options are frequently the symbols of what characterized the meaningfulness of the relationship to people. These are the aspects of the relationship that are sorely missed. Missed options are unique to the person. To an outside observer, what people identify as missed options may be easily minimized. However, identifying missed options is a way of seeing the irreversibility of the disease.

The second trigger event is known as reactivation—the process of being aware of thoughts, feelings, and sensations reminiscent of those that occurred earlier in the disease. One patient described the process of reactivation:

> I'll never forget that pain. Ever have a charley horse cramp in your leg? How would you like to have one over your entire body for 24 hours a day. That's what it felt like . . . even now when I get a minor leg cramp, boy, I go back to the first time so quickly . . .

Reactivation enables the person to see that his or her reality has changed. There is a difference from then to now.

Once the person and the family acknowledge the disease, there is still the need to be aware of the consequences of the disease and its impact on their lives. The process of becoming aware and of making changes that are supportive of the person's and the family's expectations, as well as self and family perception, is inherent in the life transition. The purpose of becoming aware is to move from a position of unknown but changed circumstances to a position of being able to redefine the circumstances. The intrinsic function of these processes is to have the person become aware and to create meaning in his or her changed circumstances, and thus to begin to construct a new reality.

As previously stated, once people acknowledge the irreversibility of the disease, uncertainty is reduced. At this time, additional information is no longer useful. The person no longer seeks more information about the reasons for the diagnosis, no longer examines the events surrounding the initial diagnosis and treatment, no longer seeks absolute cures, and no longer seeks answers to what went wrong. It is helpful to recall that, initially, the information reduced uncertainty because it gave the person a means to explain or understand what had happened. The notion that "The more information I have the more control I have" is the basis for the information-seeking behavior. The initial expectation of the person is that information alone will reduce uncertainty. To some extent, it does reduce uncertainty in the beginning. However, as the person becomes aware of the consequences of the disease, uncertainty again increases.

As the patient and the family recognize that the person is not going to "break out of it," and no "new medicine" is being discovered, uncertainty increases. Uncertainty also increases with the many complications and instructions that impact the patient's and family's daily living and relationships. Uncertainty increases as people realize the implications of ESRD and long term dialysis. The patients and families reduced this uncertainty by engaging in processes described as comparative testing, normalization, and minimizing missed options. These processes further enable the person to progress and structure a new reality.

Comparative testing is a process in which one measures oneself against an identified model, noting similarities and differences. Subjects in this study described the process. A son of one of the patients used comparative testing to reduce his uncertainty about his father's disease. He said, "I've got a friend who was in Vietnam and he's on dialysis. He's got dialysis plus he's got diabetes real bad. He's going blind." Later, he said, "For us, dad's disease isn't that great of an illness. Like my daughter — she's got a friend with no arms or legs and she goes to high school. Her situation is a lot worse than a lot of people . . . She copes . . . She is more handicapped than my father."

Another patient said, "There are guys who have bigger problems than I do. Look at the problems they have and I only got this. They got diabetes, half of their legs off and they got kidney trouble besides."

All subjects reported engaging in some means of comparative testing that reduced uncertainty. All subjects also reported experiencing normalization. Normalization is described as behaving in ways that mirror the standards established by the core society. One spouse reported,

> . . . He did not like us always pampering him and taking the phone off the hook, so he wouldn't be bothered . . . he wanted to be more of a normal part of the family. He did not want us to intercept the grandchildren's visits or anything . . . if it got too bad, he would just go off to bed if he felt he couldn't take it. I think that treating them normally is pretty important.

Another said, "Our daughter was a nurse and she would say all the time, 'Oh that's normal — all patients do that.' It was easier knowing he was normal."

Finally, a way that persons deal with ESRD is to minimize the impact of the disease and missed options. One spouse said, "We're going to take a trip starting Saturday. We're going to Kansas City. It's just going to take a little arranging with dialysis, we're able to do that. You have to do a little modification of things, but it can be done." Minimizing missed options involves using strategies that lessen, substitute, delay, and redefine behavior a person once claimed as his or her own. These processes reduce the uncertainty that family and patients report experiencing.

For example, two patients reported they could no longer play golf. One felt it was too much trouble and simply said, "The hell with it." Another patient said she rode along on a golf cart with her son and watched others play the game. Both patients minimized their missed options, but in different ways.

In summary, all subjects in this study described engaging in comparative testing, normalization, and minimizing missed options. Subjects were noted to be engaged at different points in the transition. Uncertainty was reduced for all subjects. The study, in addition to confirming the processes of life transition theory, gives rise to other interesting findings. For example, there were incongruencies between the husband and wife responses. This disparity was especially noted in perceptions of the marital relationship and the patterns of communication. For instance, the wife would report that the husband got mad whether she reminded him of his medications or not. She said, "I can't win . . . I gotta turn the other cheek." Further, she said, "He doesn't talk to me about how he feels. I wish he would." In contrast, the husband said, "My wife is very supportive. I wouldn't know what to do without her." Regarding communication he said, "I tell her." Later he said, "It doesn't bother me to talk about things." It is unknown if these discrepancies in the subjects' responses existed prior to the disease's onset or evolved in response to the disease.

The second finding, which is consistent with other research findings, was that two of the spouses experienced physical problems following the diagnosis and the initiation of dialysis for their husbands. Both women were able to make the connection between their physical symptomatology and the stress on them as a result of their spouses' illness.

Not surprisingly, the adult children living at home were more engaged in their fathers' disease process than adult children not living at home. For instance, one woman said, "I call my brother and I say 'Mark, you don't know what it's like,' and he says, 'I know, I know, I know,' but I know they just don't understand."

In contrast, an adult child living outside the family home said,

". . . it's just the way it goes. I don't think it's changed anybody's way of life except my mother's. There is not much you can do."

The length of the illness and time on dialysis varied from patient to patient. Generally, the subjects from the families with the longest history of illness reported more processes that indicated progress toward incorporating or integrating the disease and structuring a new reality than those subjects who had had an ill member for a one-year period. The latter family reported, "He's going to come out of this and start feeling better." The pattern of that family said, "I shall feel that I'll get better." Whereas, the patient who had the disease the longest reported, "Oh, it isn't tragic to me. It's a pain in the neck is what it is. It's not tragic, we'll live through it."

Lastly, in this study, subjects were asked to complete the Family APGAR questionnaire. Interestingly, the family average score suggested a highly functional group. The patient subjects rated their families with the highest score, the adult children reported the lowest scores and all three spouses rated their families the same.

In conclusion, this study utilized the life transition theory to describe family responses to an adult member diagnosed with end-stage renal disease and receiving hemodialysis treatments.

Uncertainty was manifested by all subjects. The sources of uncertainty were reported. Subjects engaged in processes that were described as reducing uncertainty.

This study was a first attempt to use the theory to study family responses rather than only the individual responding to his/her disrupted reality.

A significant variation was noted in the marital dyad's perception of patterns, and in those adult children living outside the immediate family environment. Further, the adult children seemed to be engaged in multiple transitions. These findings warrant further inquiry. It would be useful to further explore where the transitions of the members interface and relate, which have priority, and why some may take precedence over others.

Families Coping
with the Multiple Crises
of Chronic Illness

Maria J. Paluszny
Martin M. DeBeukelaer
William A. Rowane

The decreased incidence of acute infectious diseases and advances in the treatment of chronic disease have increased the lifespan of children with chronic illness (Stein and Jessop 1984). The number of children in the United States afflicted with chronic disease or other permanent physical handicaps is now estimated to be greater than 2 million (Gliedman and Roth 1980), with an overall incidence of approximately 5 to 10 percent during the childhood period (Perrin and Gerrity 1984). It has been estimated that 20 to 30 percent of this group have experienced significant psychological or behavioral difficulties some time during their childhood or adolescence (Lavigne and Burns 1981).

There is great stress and limitation on the chronically ill child or adolescent, especially in light of ongoing developmental issues, making his or her coping tasks more difficult. Fears of abandonment, separation, and those fears associated with various medical procedures are more manifest in younger children (Rae-Grant, 1985), while adolescent concerns about changing body image, developing self-identity, ambivalence about continuing dependence

Maria J. Paluszny, MD, is affiliated with the Department of Psychiatry, Medical College of Ohio, Toledo, OH. Martin M. DeBeukelaer, MD, is Director of Pediatric Nephrology, and is Associate Professor of Pediatrics, Division of Nephrology, Department of Pediatrics, Medical College of Ohio, Toledo, OH. William A. Rowane, MD, is Fellow in Child Psychiatry, Medical College of Ohio, Toledo, OH.

on parents and other caretakers (Gunther 1985) and peer acceptance (Sargent and Liebman 1985) are more prominent. Renal disease in particular, with its invasive procedures and frequent hospitalizations, interferes with the normal continuity of development in the child, besides eliciting concerns of disfigurement and discomfort. One study involving children and adolescents with chronic renal disease showed delay in the development of body image and mental capacity (Trickey, White, and DeBeukelaer 1982), illustrating the disruptive nature of this illness.

There exists a significant interactive effect between illness and family, in that an ongoing illness both affects and is affected by the family situation. This is evidenced in a recent comprehensive review by Shapiro (1983). As opposed to limited acute illness, chronic illness is long and relentless, with intermittent exacerbating crises affecting both the family and the ill child. Each specific crisis elicits a bereavement response in the family, as descriptively outlined by Bicknell (1983), with the family processing through the stages of shock, panic, denial, grief, bargaining, acceptance — ego-centered, then other-centered work. The potential for a maladaptive response at any stage exists, causing family distress and dysfunction. The family continually grieves the loss of the "healthy" child, as well as dealing with discrete crises. Child developmental and family life crises will also have special impact on the family's coping capability in the context of the child's chronic illness. In childhood renal disease, a recent study showed significant family difficulties related to financial problems and the child's physical incapacitation, compared to other chronic illnesses and controls (Holroyd and Guthrie 1986).

With regard to family subsystem coping, a recent critique of the literature revealed increased marital distress in parents of chronically ill children but no significant difference in divorce rate as compared to control (Sabbeth and Leventhal 1984). Another review (Drotar and Crawford 1984) found that the presence of chronic illness may increase subjective distress and contribute to increased risk of psychosocial disturbance for siblings of the ill child.

In families having significant difficulties dealing with chronic childhood illness, family-oriented psychotherapy, in collaboration with medical management, with concomitant individual and/or marital therapy when indicated, has been found to be helpful in improving child and family functioning. One center reports significant improvement in greater than 80 percent of cases treated (Sargent and Liebman 1985). Because of the psychosocial difficulties associated with childhood renal disease and its treatments, a multitherapeutic approach in special children's centers has been recommended (Wolters 1979; Reichwald-Klugger et al. 1986).

STRATEGIC SHORT-TERM THERAPY

The pediatric nephrology team at the Medical College of Ohio consists of a pediatric nephrologist (M.M.DeB.), a renal nurse educator, a social worker, a renal dietician, and a child psychiatrist (M.J.P). A fellow in child psychiatry (W.A.R.) is currently also assigned to the team. The team follows children with a variety of renal problems including transplant patients, patients on dialysis, and children with progressively declining renal function.

From a psychiatric standpoint the basic intervention with these patients is short-term supportive therapy at strategic points during the child's illness. These strategic points can be viewed as five stages:

1. When the diagnosis is first made.
2. When decrease in renal function or increasing physical symptoms present a problem for the child and family.
3. When a life crisis occurs.
4. When development maladjustments interfere with compliance.
5. When the team and/or family recognize that little more can be done.

Time of Diagnosis

Any time a diagnosis of chronic illness is made it is a shock and a crisis for the family. Perhaps, however, the most devastating time is when the news is told to the parents of a newborn. Though chronic renal failure is rarely diagnosed in the postnatal stage, acute renal failure often is. Approximately 70 percent of instances of renal failure in the first year of life occur in the first week of life. Most of these infants have congenital anomalies of the kidneys and urinary tract and many have additional congenital anomalies.

When parents first become aware that their infant is not perfect they may have problems in bonding with the child. Winnicott (1958), Bowlby (1969), and others have shown that infants gradually develop specific attachments to their caretakers. This process is greatly enhanced by the parents' first joyous acceptance of the child. However, when a baby is imperfect the parents frequently go through a process of grief and have difficulty accepting the infant. The process of bonding is delayed and may be incomplete. One mother of an infant with congenital anomalies stated this very well when she told me, "I don't feel about her the same as I did with my other babies. There is a distance. I keep thinking, what will she be like when she is older?" This infant had a myelomeningocele and the mother was aware of the many problems possible, including the eventual renal failure that can be associated with this defect. Intervention in this type of situation is difficult, in that exploring a mother's feelings about the newborn may increase the mother's guilt and thus interfere even more with bonding. Listening to the mother and being accepting of her feelings, providing support through availability, as well as helping the mother and father support each other, is probably the most effective intervention. In this way the "mothering" the new parents receive can be translated by them into mothering the infant. Support can also be obtained through extended family. Parent association groups can be very helpful after the parents have worked through their denial and some of their grief and start planning for the future. However, in these first stages exposure to parents of children with similar and frequently more impaired infants can be overwhelming.

When the diagnosis of renal failure or another incurable chronic illness is made in an older child, the problem of bonding is not an issue. However, the parents still experience the same feelings of shock, denial, grief, guilt, and anger at life, God, and of course, professionals. The basic approach is still to help them accept the child's handicap by providing support through availability, an attentive ear, and practical suggestions.

Progressive Deterioration

The second stage for involvement is when decreasing renal function or increasing physical symptoms present a problem for the child or family. Perhaps the best way to discuss this is by describing two cases.

Case 1. Peter, a two-year-old boy and the only child in a one-parent family, had multiple admissions for problems related to progressive renal failure secondary to an obstructive uropathy. While he was maintained on peritoneal dialysis he had recurrent infections. Later he had persistent hypertension, which resulted in a stroke causing temporary partial paralysis. When a renal transplant was done Peter had clotting problems and the transplant had to be removed hours after the surgery. Throughout these crises Peter's mother remained realistically concerned but managed to provide affection as well as setting limits when necessary to get Peter to cooperate with the staff. In some ways the mother's ability to accept and deal appropriately with Peter through these various crises is surprising as the mother had a very difficult background – she ran away from home at the age of 15 to marry Peter's father and divorced him when she learned of his extramarital affairs. She remarried but her second husband was an alcoholic. A few months prior to Peter's starting his multiple hospitalizations at the Medical College of Ohio, the mother experienced several personal crises. First, her husband, Peter's father, died. She moved with her second husband to a different state, away from her family, and then, because of her second husband's drinking and abusive behavior, she separated from him just one week prior to Peter's first admission to our hospital. We may well ask how the mother could manage with so many overwhelming crises. Basically, she managed by using a variety of supports. First, her relationship to Peter was one of mutual support. She viewed Peter as the one worthwhile aspect of her life, someone who needed her and returned unquestioned love. Peter is indeed a very bright and charming little boy and even after the stroke made remarkedly rapid progress. Despite his problems he is rarely irritable, and usually happy and outgoing. The second support came from the extended family. Even though the extended family lived out of state, during each hospitalization either one of the mother's parents or her brother drove up to be with her. This extensive support for a single-parent family is unusual, as most extended families do not have such close ties or the financial resources to be so available. Finally, the mother herself was such an open and pleasant lady that all the hospital staff was eager to spend time with her. Even after discharge the mother sometimes came to the ward to just "visit old friends." In addition, the mother called me when she felt overwhelmed and was able to use suggestions and advice regarding her life and Peter very well.

Case 2. In contrast to the above case, Cheryl, a nine-year-old girl, had fewer medical problems but many more psychological difficulties. Cheryl, the older of two children from an intact family, was diagnosed as having a "prune belly" syndrome at birth. She had multiple urinary anomalies and progressive renal failure. At the age of nine she was seen prior to a renal transplant. In the evaluation Cheryl appeared to be a serious, pseudo-mature child with many concerns about school. She was having problems with her homework, which she and her mother worked on for hours each day. In addition, she was repeatedly teased by her peers, who found out she was enuretic and had to wear diapers. At times they also called her "fatso" because of her "prune belly." Because of work commitments, the father could not come for the evaluation, but the mother was very involved. At first she wanted to know if it was safe for Cheryl to wait alone in the lobby as she feared Cheryl could be kidnapped from our waiting room. In talking about Cheryl she described how professionals had told her Cheryl would never walk because of the prune belly. Nevertheless, she spent hours daily with Cheryl strengthening her muscles so that eventually Cheryl had no problems walking. She also described how she tried to help Cheryl with bedwetting. However, she could not understand why we felt it was so important to teach Cheryl to put on her own diapers. The mother insisted that she had to do this as she believed that Cheryl, despite her nine years, could not manage on her own. She described her husband as being very invested in both children and said he spent time with them when he was not working. However, she also described him as "unavailable" and gave the impression he was unavailable to her as a support. Her family lived some distance away and they rarely visited. When the issue of a kidney transplant was raised, the mother was very interested in being the donor. When therapy for Cheryl was recommended, the mother initially was reluctant but eventually agreed to have someone from school work with Cheryl regarding school and peer issues.

These two cases show very different parental acceptance of the child with renal failure and his or her problems. Peter's mother had fully accepted Peter with his handicap. She could be empathic as well as set limits for him. She used support from family and professionals effectively. Cheryl's mother, in order to maintain control over her ambivalent feelings, externalized the issue of control to other issues, even to the point of insisting on diapering Cheryl. Some anger related to Cheryl's problems was displaced to professionals, i.e., they did not know enough and said Cheryl would not walk and did not know how to handle Cheryl. However, in addition, there was some anger directed at Cheryl. This was evident by the frequent struggles over homework and the mother's angry unrealistic fears that Cheryl could be kidnapped from the waiting room. The mother was only willing to accept partial support in that she arranged therapy so that it would only be focused on school and not on her relationship with Cheryl. One wonders if her acceptance of support from her husband was also on a similar, limited basis.

Life Crises

Broadly interpreted, a life crisis may refer to any drastic change to which the patient and family must adjust. Significant changes within the family or a major change in the child's renal disease can be a life crisis. When both of these occur simultaneously, issues and reactions may be very confusing. Mark, a seven-year-old boy, was admitted for a cadaver renal transplant. His major concerns, however, were not the operation but rather the changes in his family. Mark's mother had recently separated from his father and, while the divorce was pending, moved in with another man whom Mark called his "stepdad," "other dad," or sometimes just plain "dad." Physically, Mark did very well after the transplant. His psychological reactions, however, did not parallel his physical improvement. At first Mark was eager to see all his family, including both the biological father and the mother's live-in partner. Later, Mark began to talk more about his natural father, commenting on all the wonderful gifts he brought. However, when one questioned him specifically about the gifts, Mark would occasionally refer to both men as dad, and thus it was not clear which gift came from whom. Soon Mark began to complain about his stepdad, i.e., that his stepdad drank, that he was destructive, and that sometimes he was abusive to his mother. When the mother was seen alone she said, while crying, that she still loved Mark's father and knew he loved the children, but that he was very irresponsible and frequently drank, and often after drinking he was abusive to her. She denied that her live-in partner had ever been abusive to her. When we talked with the stepfather, he appeared to be very understanding and patient with Mark. It appeared that with the prolonged hospitalization and the friendly visits with his natural father, Mark had split the images of the two fathers, with the natural father becoming the "good" father and the stepfather becoming the "bad" father. In this way the natural father fit into Mark's fantasized image. In addition, Mark possibly projected some of his anxieties and guilt related to the transplant onto his stepfather. During the hospitalization and following the transplant, Mark would not discuss the operation at all, except at one time he mentioned he got "somebody's kidney." Possibly in Mark's mind he got something that belonged to somebody else, just like the stepfather got a family that belonged to someone else. This interpretation, however, was not made. Instead we elected to wait and see how Mark would do once he was discharged from the hospital. Sometime later, the mother informed us that after returning home, Mark's relationship with his stepfather improved, returning to its usual friendly interaction. Thus Mark was able to resolve his conflict without further intervention. However, without the support and understanding of both mother and stepfather, Mark probably would not have managed so well.

Developmental Maladjustments

Compliance may be a problem at any age. However, we frequently see this problem in our adolescent group with renal failure. Adolescents typically attempt to achieve independence by struggling with their parents for power and control. When a life-threatening illness makes the adolescent feel more vulnerable, the struggle is more intense. Jane, a 15-year-old girl with a myelomeningocele, was admitted because of progressive renal problems. During the hospitalization we learned that Jane did not catheterize herself according to schedule. Jane came from a reconstituted family: her stepfather was several years younger than her mother and only ten years older than Jane. Jane's overdetermined hostility and rejection of her stepfather indicated a possible defense against an attraction to the man. Later we learned the mother worked full time and the stepfather took care of Jane and the other children. In addition, it was he who reminded Jane when she should catheterize. His insistence on being in control was as intense as Jane's rejection of him. The obvious sexual undertones were covered by hostility on both sides. In trying to approach the stepfather on an intellectual level, we got nowhere. He was already threatened by seeing himself as a "househusband," and to give up any control was unthinkable. We then attempted to work with Jane. Jane was somewhat resistant to seeing a "shrink" but she was captive, because other medical problems forced her to remain in the hospital for seven weeks. The work with Jane was focused on independence and taking control of her body. When family issues came up, no interpretation was attempted regarding Jane's possible attraction to her stepfather. Rather, we emphasized the stepfather's role as mother's husband. Likewise, wherever possible, Jane's interaction with male peers was stressed. By the time Jane left there was still anger at her stepfather but the intensity was greatly diminished. Jane was more independent, was looking forward to going to a new school, and was more outgoing and friendly. In particular she appeared to be interested in boys on the ward and was flirtatious with the male medical students. It appeared that we had been successful in decreasing some of the ambivalent attraction of Jane to her stepfather and in helping Jane with appropriate male peer relations.

Terminal Crisis or Event

There is only one thing more difficult than breaking the news to parents that the child has a chronic illness, and that one thing is telling them that nothing else can be done. The child with end-stage renal disease who is no longer a candidate for a transplant, and for whom dialysis and other supportive measures are no longer effective, represents this rare category of patients. Often this stage is similar to the first stage, when the parents are first told of the illness: denial, hope for a miracle, anger at professionals, and guilt may again be the parents' reaction. To make matters worse, professionals often have difficulty in handling their own feelings and are thus less available psychologically to give support to the parents. Dan, a six-year-old boy who was terminally ill, illustrates some of these reactions. Dan had become extremely ill once before but had a remarkable remission. After being home one month he was back again and appeared terminal. His parents had two other children. The father and grandparents took care of these two children while the mother stayed in the hospital day and night. Occasionally she stayed at the Ronald McDonald House (a residential setting for parents with inpatient children) but most of the time she was in the hospital. The nursing staff found the mother very difficult. She seemed to be demanding nursing staff's time for herself. She would spend more time with staff or other patients' parents than with Dan. In addition, she kept saying that he would again improve, despite his continued downhill course.

When regular meetings were set up with the mother, it became clear that she had problems even before the current crisis. She had a history of depression and psychiatric hospitalizations. She felt her husband had never been very supportive of her and at times felt worthless. Basically, the short-term intervention consisted of letting the mother ventilate and making some practical suggestions to her. Suggestions were aimed at getting the mother to see her other children more, to get the father more involved, and to intervene between the mother and the other professionals. Before Dan died the mother was going home at regular intervals while the father stayed with Dan. While in the hospital she spent time holding Dan rather than visiting with staff and patients. The nursing staff and physicians found her easier to deal with and no longer avoided her.

CONCLUSION

In each of the five stages we intervene with families by providing support on a short-term basis. In addition, whenever necessary, we mediate between staff and families to increase understanding. The tactic is not to make interpretations of defenses but rather to strengthen the family's and child's own coping devices. On the one hand, by increasing the child's and family's acceptance of the physical problem, we aim to prevent disillusionment through unrealistic expectations. On the other hand, by preventing unnecessary overprotection, we aim to promote appropriate separation and developmental progress. We believe this approach is effective with most of our families.

REFERENCES

Bicknell, J. 1983. "The Psychopathology of Handicap" *British Journal of Medical Psychology* 56:167-168.

Bowlby, J. 1969. *Attachment and Loss*. Vol 1. London: Hogarth Press.

Drotar, D. and P. Crawford. 1984. "Psychological Adaptation of Siblings of Chronically Ill Children: Research, Practice and Implications." *Developmental Health and Behavioral Pediatrics* 6:355-362.

Gliedman, J. and W. Roth. 1980. *The Unexpected Minority – Handicapped Children in America*. New York: Harcourt, Brace Jovanovich.

Gunther, M. 1985. "Acute Onset Serious Chronic Organic Illness in Adolescence: Some Critical Issues." *Adolescent Psychiatry* 12:59-76.

Holroyd, J. and D. Guthrie. 1986. "Family Stress with Chronic Childhood Illness: Cystic Fibrosis Neuromuscular Disease and Renal Disease." *Journal of Clinical Psychology* 42(4):552-561.

Lavigne J. and W. Burns. 1981. *Pediatric Psychology: An Introduction for Pediatricians and Psychologists*. New York: Grune and Stratton.

Perrin, E. and P. Gerrity. 1984. "Development of Children with a Chronic Illness." *Pediatric Clinics of North America* 31:19-31.

Rae-Grant, Q. 1985. "Psychological Problems in the Medically Ill Child." *Psychiatric Clinics of North America* 85(4):653-663.

Reichwald-Klugger, E., K. Weck, R. Korn et al. 1986. "Psychosocial Adaptation of Children and Their Parents to Hospital and Home Hemodialysis." *Dialysis and Transplantation* 15(8):453-459.

Sabbeth, B. and J. Leventhal. 1984. Marital Adjustment to Chronic Childhood Illness: A Critique of the Literature. *Pediatrics* 73(6):762-768.

Sargent, J. and R. Liebman. 1985. "Childhood Chronic Illness: Issues for Psychotherapists." *Community Mental Health Journal* 21(4):294-311.

Shapiro, J. 1983. "Family Reactions and Coping Strategies in Response to the Physically Ill or Handicapped Child: A Review." *Social Science in Medicine* 17(14):913-931.

Stein, R. and D. Jessop. 1984. "Does Pediatric Home Care Make a Difference for Children with Chronic Illness? Findings from the Pediatric Ambulatory Care Treatment Study." *Pediatrics* 73(6):845-853.

Trickey, B., J. White, M. DeBeukelaer. 1982. "A Study of the Body Image with

Chronic Renal Failure." *Physical and Occupational Therapy in Pediatrics* 1(4):35-44.

Winnicott, D. 1958. *Through Pediatrics to Psychoanalysis*. London: Tavistock.

Wolters, W. 1979. "Psychosocial Care at a Center for Hemodialysis and Renal Transplantation in Children and Adolescents." *Acta Paedopsychiatrie* 44:85-89.

Is Ignorance Bliss?
ESRD Patients' Reactions
to the Question
of Spousal Fidelity

Kathleen Degen

The professional literature is replete with studies of the prevalence and type of sexual dysfunction in ESRD patients. Less has been published regarding the incidence of divorce or marital dissolution through separation. No information could be found on patient reactions to the questions of spousal fidelity.

Throughout the last two decades, profound changes in mores and morals have modified societal views on fidelity in marriage. Two decades ago, marital fidelity was considered a societal norm. Movies, television, and written representations overtly supported the concept of monogamy. Infidelity was not openly advocated or touted as a desirable way of living, nor was infidelity presented as a valid way of dealing with intramarital problems, economic or otherwise.

We do have some evidence of a bipartite or double standard, however. That is, "lip service" to fidelity or portrayal of a public image of fidelity was the norm, while covertly, if kept quiet, sexual liaisons outside marriage went on without family or societal disapproval. Evidence for this view can be found in the Kinsey report (1948). This work investigated, by questionnaire, the prevalence of extramarital sexual activity among married men and women. Sixty percent of married men, and 40 percent of married women, admit-

Kathleen Degen, MD, is Assistant Clinical Professor of Psychiatry, College of Physicians and Surgeons, Columbia University, St. Luke's-Roosevelt Medical Center, New York, NY.

27

ted to extramarital affairs. Infidelity occurred, unlike the ideal depicted in the TV shows "The Ozzie and Harriet Show" or "Father Knows Best." A recent TV serial, "All in the Family," shows Archie, a married father, express interest in an adulterous relationship to satisfy needs unmet in his marriage or to relieve feelings about intrafamily conflict. Similarly, "Country Girl," a film of the 1940s, depicts a woman married to an emotionally sick husband who contemplates an affair that would commence after she "left" her husband. In contrast, recent films, such as "Diary of a Mad Housewife," demonstrate a guiltless extramarital liaison sought by the protagonist as a refuge from her emotionally troubled husband.

Whether actual practice in real life has been altered is not known. However, the erosion of the former cultural ideals of the lifelong, monogamous commitment of marriage is reflected in changed media representations. These ever more powerful and ubiquitous media portrayals are telling us that adultery is a legitimate alternative to cope with the suffering of a panoply of intramarital problems from unsatisfactory sex to absent praise, lack of love, or modified physical appearance.

ESRD patients experience deteriorating sexual function, energy, physical appearance, and reduced ability to show love by meeting other, nonsexual needs of spouses. Their marriages are fraught with the likelihood of marital problems. ESRD patients are, like us, exposed to media messages telling them that infidelity is a valid choice for dissatisfied partners. Do ESRD patients express feelings on the question of spousal fidelity?

In this investigation, three specific questions relating to fidelity are asked, with special attention to the question of whether a patient wishes to know of the indiscretion, should adultery occur.

METHOD

Information on ESRD patients' concerns about spousal fidelity was gathered from five men and one woman who were part of a sexual dysfunction study. Another woman was subsequently added to comprise a total study group of seven ESRD patients. There was no control group.

The subjects were chosen by patient interest in participating and by staff perception of the patient's reliability to keep the designated appointment and to answer questions truthfully.

All seven patients were married or had a committed partner. The word "spouse" is used to mean committed partner, legally married or not. All participants had been on dialysis for at least 13 years. The questions, asked by an interviewer, were:

1. Do you think your spouse/committed partner is faithful?
2. If your spouse were not faithful, would you want to know?
3. Would you feel comfortable with the unfaithfulness of your spouse?

The questions were asked to evoke "yes" or "no" responses. However, other patient reactions were noted.

RESULTS

Five male (N = 5) and one female (N = 2) answered in the affirmative to "Do you think your spouse is faithful?" The woman who answered no to the question said, additionally, that while she thought her husband was having an affair, she was not sure, because he was discreet. Also, she mentioned that he continued to bring home his paycheck and treat her the same as before she became ill. She attributed his possible extramarital affair to her inability to have sex with him. Her desire for sex was inhibited, and she had no energy to "go places with him."

All seven patients responded negatively to query #2: "If your spouse were not faithful, would you want to know?" One male (N = 5) and one female (N = 2) responded affirmatively to question #3: "Would you feel comfortable with the unfaithfulness of your spouse?" The male affirming comfort with spousal infidelity gave as his reason his inability to satisfy his wife sexually due to intractable erectile dysfunction. He did not worry about losing her to another, as he felt their love for each other was very strong and would keep them together. The female affirmative mentioned, as noted earlier, that her husband, whom she suspected of having an affair but would not want to know for sure, continued to treat her as before her illness, and did not flaunt his affair.

DISCUSSION

ESRD patients were asked three questions to assess their reactions to the issue of spousal fidelity. The results raised more questions, yet several points became clear. First, I would like to focus on the way patients responded to the questions.

It was clear from this investigation that all the patients studied had conscious thoughts and feelings, or preconscious thoughts and feelings that were easily evoked, about the faithfulness of their mate. For example, although only one woman suspected her partner of adultery, she asserted that she did not want to know for certain.

It was also clear that, despite documentation by multiple studies of ESRD patients being out of touch with feelings, all the patients answered the questions without hesitation and were able to elaborate on their responses without effort. The patients' ease in expressing complex and emotionally charged feelings suggests the importance of the issue of spousal fidelity to them. In a similar vein, I would speculate that ESRD patients can access thoughts and feelings if questioned about matters of emotional importance to them.

In much of the professional literature, ESRD patients have been presented as largely "alexithymic" or bereft of conscious fantasies and feelings. This overt alexithymic presentation may be a mask, due more to lack of motivation to answer health care providers' questions about issues of little emotional importance to them than to absent fantasy life. Typically, the ESRD patient has been asked questions over and over—questions such as, "Are you taking your medicine?", "Are you following your diet?" Redundancy and absence of emotional bonding with the interviewer in a meaningful way may induce boredom and a sense of futility. As one patient put it, "Always the same questions. What difference does it make? I always feel the same . . . ." I suggest that asking questions of more universal human importance would establish a crucial emotional bond with the ESRD patient. This bond would serve as a catalyst to reduce the compartmentalization of fantasies and feelings. I maintain that for many there is compartmentalization rather than true alexithymia.

Another aspect of patients' lack of motivation to access feelings in response to care providers' inquiry is the "them/us" division. The patients are "them," and the providers are "us." This separatism has categorical convenience. Yet, the categories imply that one label is better than the other, unlike the categories "apples" and "oranges" or "horses" and "zebras." Distance is thereby created between us and our patients. One way of relieving the built-in tension of dichotomous thinking is to devise an inquiry that emphasizes our similarities rather than our differences, uses simple English words, and includes questions that stem from universal human concerns. To make the point clearer in the context of this essay, who among us has never worried about spousal fidelity?

In response to question #1, six patients said that they believed their spouse was faithful, perhaps reflecting a common thought that catastrophe can befall "anyone but me." A form of denial may have been involved in the responses to question #1. However, staff who knew the patients' spouses corroborated the patients' impression. As previously noted, the patient who doubted her husband's fidelity did not want to know for certain.

All seven patients would not want to know if there were an extramarital affair. The unanimous reluctance to know was an unexpected finding. The wish not to know could be classified as a subtype of denial. Professional literature and clinical observations detail the importance of denial to ESRD patients in coping with a multifaceted, chronic illness. The wish to deny an affair, should the indiscretion occur, is likely an effort, conscious or unconscious, to protect themselves from another harsh reality over which, like their illness, they feel helpless.

Two patients would feel comfortable with a spousal affair, as long as they did not know for sure. The five patients who said they would not feel comfortable with their spouse having an extramarital sexual relationship expressed concern about possible loss of the partner to the paramour.

Is ignorance bliss? Since most of the patients (5) preferred that adulterous activity not take place, ignorance was not exactly bliss, but close to it. Ideal bliss was found in perceived actual fidelity. Yet, all seven patients preferred ignorance to the unwanted knowledge of an adulterous relationship.

REFERENCE

Kinsey, A. C., W. B. Pomeroy, and C. E. Martin. 1948. *Sexual Behavior in the Human Male*. Philadelphia: W. B. Saunders Co.

Marital and Family Characteristics of Home and Hospital Dialysis Patients

Stewart Page
Mark B. Weisberg

As illustrated in recent reviews by Binik (1983) and by Weisberg and Page (1988; in press), end-stage renal disease (ESRD) has been long neglected by researchers concerned with psychological or social factors in illness.

As described by Weisberg and Page, such disease is, however, a major health problem. According to Cummings (1970), more than 50,000 persons die annually from kidney disease in the United States alone. While dialysis, the removal of toxins and excess fluid from the system, is the most common form of treatment for ESRD,

Stewart Page, PhD, is Professor of Clinical Psychology, Department of Psychology, University of Windsor, Ontario, Canada. Mark B. Weisberg, PhD, is in private practice in Psychology, Minneapolis, MN.

The present study is based, in part, upon a doctoral dissertation submitted by the first author to the Department of Psychology, University of Windsor, Windsor, Ontario.

Complete descriptions or copies of materials used in the present study are available upon request, or may be found in Weisberg (1984). Also, several analyses concerning choice of the various dialysis submodalities (i.e., home hemodialysis, home IPD, home CAPD, hospital hemodialysis, hospital IPD) not reported herein are also available upon request.

Requests for reprints should be sent to Dr. Mark B. Weisberg, 5128 Zenith Ave., Minneapolis, MN 55410.

The authors wish to acknowledge the assistance of Drs. Kevin Moreland, Catherine Green, William Balance, Robert Fehr, and Sidney Baskin in various phases of this research, as well as the staff of the Kidney Unit, Mount Carmel Mercy Hospital, Detroit, MI.

its effectiveness remains limited by the fact that development of its technical aspects has grown faster than has understanding of its psychological aspects and ramifications. Kidney disease seriously disrupts the lives of patients and their families, sexually, socially, and financially, hence the need for investigation of psychological factors that might enhance or impede adjustment to a dialysis regimen. ESRD patients undergoing dialysis treatment encounter several broad areas of stress (De-Nour 1981; Weisberg 1984). These include physiological fluctuation, deterioration, and discomfort, as well as strict dietary restrictions. With a life-threatening chronic illness, patients must also confront such issues as their mortality, fear of death, and, in fact, fear of life (Beard and Sampson 1981). The presence of serious emotional and psychological turmoil in ESRD patients has thus precipitated development of the field of psychonephrology, the study of psychological factors in dialysis and transplantation (see Drees and Gallagher 1981).

HEMODIALYSIS AND PERITONEAL DIALYSIS

In hemodialysis, the most frequent form of dialysis, blood is passed through a cleansing system to remove toxins and excess fluid. The blood is filtered through semipermeable membranes in the dialyzing machine, thus removing water, salt, and waste products. Access to the circulatory system is usually through an arteriovenous fistula. This procedure must be used an average of two or three days weekly. It may be done, however, either in the patient's home or in a hospital setting. In the former type, the patient works with spouse or partner in using, monitoring, and operating the equipment correctly. A training period is necessary. In the latter type, the patient receives the treatment passively, with hospital staff monitoring details of machine maintenance and operation, as well as monitoring blood pressure, fluid, and chemical levels. Both home and hospital hemodialysis patients must also learn the necessary medical and dietary restrictions.

An alternative treatment is peritoneal dialysis, in which no blood is removed from the body. Tubing is inserted just inside the peritoneum (the sac surrounding the abdomen), and dialysate fluid is introduced through the tubing into the peritoneum, causing dialysis of water and waste material to occur through the peritoneal sac. Fluid and waste are later drained through the same tubing. There are two commonly used forms of peritoneal dialysis. Intermittent peritoneal dialysis (IPD) can be performed either in the patient's home or in hospital. If performed at home, both patient and partner require special training in proper use of the required equipment. Another option for home peritoneal patients is continuous ambulatory peritoneal dialysis (CAPD), which functions similarly to IPD but on a continuous (24-hour) basis. In this procedure, the patient is essentially free to do normal activities while dialyzing continuously by means of a portable dialysate container. Although there are disadvantages to CAPD treatment, there are fewer nutritional and dietary restrictions than with other procedures. Both hemodialysis and peritoneal dialysis appear equally effective physiologically; detailed descriptions of these procedures are found in sources such as Friedman (1978) and Weisberg (1984).

More critical than the distinction between the various treatment procedures, for present purposes, was the issue of whether the treatment is experienced in one's home or in a hospital. The choice of whether to dialyze in hospital or at home has physiological, psychological, and economic ramifications, both for ESRD patients and medical ESRD staff. At present, however, little is known, and almost no empirical data have been gathered about family and marital factors enhancing or inhibiting success with these different modalities, or about how such factors are related to patient progress and satisfaction with the modality chosen. ESRD staff, for example, frequently see patients with equivalent degrees of organ pathology and physiological deterioration, who nevertheless show considerable variability in their response to ESRD treatment. Greater understanding of this process would be of considerable practical and medical value to these staff. Personality or other differences between those adjusting better to hospital or to home dialysis have been claimed (e.g., Lowry and Atchison 1980), but again almost no studies have been able to gather empirical data on such an issue directly from ESRD patients themselves.

The present study, therefore, studied the relationship between marital and family functioning and adjustment, on the one hand, and the choice between home and hospital dialysis on the other.

Using the Family Environment Scale and Marital Attitude Evaluation Scale (described below), data from both home and hospital patients were gathered. Data were also gathered from the spouses or partners of these patients. Aside from studying the characteristics of those choosing to dialyze in home or in hospital, some additional measures of patients' overall satisfaction and perceived efficacy of the dialysis procedures, described below, were also examined.

METHOD

Subjects

Forty-two patients of the Kidney Unit at Mt. Carmel Mercy Hospital, Detroit, participated as subjects, as did 37 partners. Most of the common renal diagnoses were represented, both in the home and hospital dialysis samples. Such diagnoses included glomerulonephritis, pyelonephritis, hypertensive renal failure, polycystic renal failure, and nephrosclerosis. Mean age for the total sample was 48.42 years for patients and 42.18 years for partners. Twenty-nine patients were female, 14 were male. Mean length of time on dialysis at the time of the study was 18.21 months. Most patients earned $10,000 or less annually, and had at least a high school education; 80 percent were unemployed, full time, at the time of the study. Also, 65 percent of the patients' partners were unemployed. Forty-three percent of the partners were spouses, with the remainder being sons, daughters, siblings, parents, or friends.

Chi-square tests indicated no significant differences between the home and hospital patients in income, marital status, number of available persons, or employment status. A t-test indicated that the hospital group (M = 55.75 yrs.) was significantly older than the home group (M = 41.77 yrs.), t(40) = 3.74, p < .006. All analyses, reported in the *Results* section below, were therefore performed with patient age as a covariate. In all cases, the obtained p levels for these analyses remained as reported below. Both groups had been determined by the unit's medical staff to be comparable in overall medical status, apart from ESRD symptoms. Three patients in each group were diabetic. It should be noted also that the use of home versus hospital dialysis was primarily a result of the patient's own decision, and not of medical or other factors. It was the policy of the Mt. Carmel Kidney Unit staff to present new ESRD patients with complete verbal and written descriptions of both home and hospital dialysis procedures, including the known advantages and disadvantages of each, from which patients freely chose their preferred modality.

Procedure

Eligible patients were contacted initially by letter, and then by telephone. All completed a form acknowledging free and informed consent for participation. The Family Environment Scale (FES) and Marital Attitudes Evaluation Scale (MATE) were completed, by appointment, at the Kidney Unit, Mt. Carmel Mercy Hospital, Detroit, under supervision of the first author. Certain demographic and medical information was also obtained from patient charts.

Patients and partners also completed several personality measures, the results of which have been reported in Weisberg and Page (1988, in press), as well as several Likert-type rating scales assessing marital and family cohesiveness as well as the degree of satisfaction with ongoing treatment. Some results involving these latter scales are presented, where relevant to the focus of the present study, in the *Results* and *Discussion* sections below.

Measures of Marital and Family Characteristics

The FES (Moos and Moos 1981) is a 100-item self-report scale, using a true-false format. The respondent describes his or her family on three basic aspects: a relationship dimension, a personal growth dimension, and a system maintenance dimension. The FES has yielded useful information in previous research concerning depression (e.g., Wetzel and Raymond 1980), alcoholism (e.g., Filstead 1979), and in the context of outcome measures in family-oriented treatment procedures (e.g., Rasmussen 1980). The relationship dimensions contain items which assess family cohesion (degree of commitment, help, and support), expressiveness (extent of encouragement to express feelings in the family), and conflict (degree of openly expressed anger and conflict). The personal growth dimensions assess independence (extent to which family members make their own decisions), achievement orientation (extent of encouragement in school and work activities), intellectual/cultural orientation (extent of encouragement of cultural, political, and intellectual activities), active/recreational orientation (support of physical activities), and a moral/religious orientation (extent of emphasis on moral or ethical matters). The system maintenance dimensions assess organization (extent to which structure and planning are stressed in the family), and control (extent to which rules and procedures are stressed).

The MATE evaluates several dimensions of intimate, close relationships and is taken from Schutz's (1978) FIRO-B scale. The MATE contains 45 items to which the subject responds using a six-point scale for each. The scale measures the degree of satisfaction and sensitivity a respondent feels toward someone, such as a spouse or partner, who is involved in an intimate relationship with the respondent. The basic dimensions of the MATE concern inclusion behavior (e.g., wanting to be given more attention by one's partner), inclusion feelings (wishing one's partner to be more interested, to feel more strongly toward one), control behavior (e.g., wanting one's partner to give one more freedom or more independence), control feelings (e.g., wishing one's partner to have more respect for one's ability to do things well), and affection (e.g., wanting one's partner to show more love and affection toward the respondent). Responses are made to each MATE item from two perspectives: "I want you to . . ." (type I responses) and "I feel that you want me to . . ." (type II responses). The MATE was used in the present study in order to examine patterns of satisfaction in both the home and hospital dialysis samples, as well as to examine any differences in patterns of response between the two treatment modalities. Both patients and partners completed the FES and MATE scales. Complete descriptions of all scales used are presented in Weisberg (1984).

RESULTS

FES Results, Home and Hospital Samples

The mean scores and standard deviations for all home and hospital patients and partners, on the MATE and FES scales, are presented in Tables 1 and 2.

With the choice of home versus hospital dialysis as the nominal (classification) variable, and with the ten FES subscales serving as dependent variable measures, a multivariate analysis of variance (MANOVA), using the Statistical Analysis System Institute's SAS (1985) GLM (General Linear Models) procedure, was performed on the patients' responses. The resulting multivariate F value was significant, $F(10, 31) = 2.17$, $p < .04$, using the Hotelling-Lawley Trace Test criterion. Univariate F (ANOVA) tests were then performed, as well as a discriminant function analysis, using the SAS (1985) STEPDISC procedure, in which the choice of home versus hospital dialysis served as the classification variable. The STEPDISC procedure selects predictor variables which still contribute discriminating power, at $F \leq .15$, after adjusting for their correlation with other potential predictor variables. Two subscales were entered as the most discriminating predictors by the stepwise procedure, namely, family expressiveness, $F(1, 40) = 9.37$, $p < .004$, and the patient active/recreational subscale, $F(1, 40) = 7.32$, $p < .01$.

With the choice of home versus hospital dialysis as the nominal variable, as above, a MANOVA was also performed for the partners' data. The multivariate F was significant, $F(10, 26) = 3.47$, $p < .005$, using the Hotelling-Lawley Trace Test criterion. Again using the home versus hospital choice as the classification variable, a stepwise discriminant function analysis, using the STEPDISC procedure, was then performed, using the FES subscales as predictor variables. The stepwise procedure identified the expressiveness subscale as the best predictor of dialysis modality, $F(1, 36) = 9.54$, $p < .004$; then cohesion, $F(1, 36) = 7.11$, $p < .01$; then conflict, $F(1, 36) = 3.74$, $p < .06$; then independence, $F(1, 36) = 2.74$, $p < .10$; then control, $F(1, 36) = 3.48$, $p < .07$; and then intellectual/cultural orientation, $F(1, 36) = 2.71$, $p < .11$.

TABLE 1. FES and MATE Scores for Patients Dialyzing at Home, and Partners

	Patients		Partners	
FES subscale	M	SD	M	SD
Cohesion	7.14	2.01	7.40	1.85
Conflict	2.18	1.87	1.20	1.17
Expressiveness	6.09	2.02	6.15	1.87
Independence	6.86	1.32	6.30	1.34
Achievement	6.05	1.13	5.40	2.04
Intell-Cult.	6.32	2.38	5.60	1.88
Active-Recr.	4.77	1.90	4.85	1.73
Moral-Relig.	6.59	2.06	6.60	2.09
Organizat.	5.82	2.11	5.80	2.69
Control	4.45	2.09	4.05	1.82
MATE subscale	M	SD	M	SD
Incl. Behav. I	3.95	3.03	2.11	2.08
Incl. Behav. II	3.00	2.71	3.11	2.56
Incl. Feel. I	4.25	3.19	2.63	2.36
Incl. Feel. II	3.65	3.03	3.05	2.78
Contr. Behav. I	3.90	2.63	2.79	2.97
Contr. Behav. II	4.40	2.82	2.79	2.97
Contr. Feel. I	5.00	3.28	3.05	3.21
Contr. Feel. II	5.00	2.88	3.47	3.34
Affection I	3.80	3.43	2.16	2.52
Affection II	3.15	3.38	3.16	3.08

TABLE 2. FES and MATE Scores for Patients Dialyzing in Hospital, and Partners

	Patients		Partners	
FES subscale	M	SD	M	SD
Cohesion	7.30	1.26	7.60	1.25
Expressiveness	4.50	1.24	4.53	1.18
Conflict	2.00	1.21	2.59	1.54
Independence	6.85	1.53	7.00	1.37
Achievement	6.40	1.10	6.00	1.37
Intell./Cult.	6.00	1.56	5.82	1.51
Active/Recrea.	5.95	1.57	5.47	1.55
Moral/Relig.	7.60	1.43	7.24	1.09
Organiz.	6.70	1.45	6.53	1.23
Control	5.60	1.05	5.71	1.40
MATE subscale	M	SD	M	SD
Incl. Beh. I	5.28	2.44	2.13	2.28
Incl. Beh. II	4.72	2.40	3.13	1.41
Incl. Feel. I	6.33	2.38	3.50	2.22
Incl. Feel. II	6.44	2.64	4.88	1.89
Cont. Beh. I	5.72	2.02	4.19	2.26
Cont. Beh. II	6.39	2.23	4.75	2.14
Cont. Feel. I	7.67	1.68	5.88	2.16
Cont. Feel. II	7.17	2.53	3.75	2.29
Affection I	6.28	2.93	4.19	2.40
Affection II	6.56	3.05	6.11	2.11

MATE Results, Home and Hospital Samples

With the choice of home versus hospital dialysis as the nominal variable, and with the ten MATE subscales as the dependent variable measures, a MANOVA was performed, first using data obtained from patients. The obtained multivariate F, using the Hotelling-Lawley Trace criterion, was nonsignificant; however, a stepwise discriminant function analysis, with home versus hospital choice as the classification variable, showed that the affection subscale (type II) did discriminate significantly between the two modalities, $F(1, 33) = 10.58$, $p < .002$.

Regarding the data obtained from partners, a MANOVA, with home versus hospital choice as the nominal variable, was significant, $F(10,24) = 3.51$, $p < .005$, using the Hotelling-Lawley Trace criterion. Further univariate (ANOVA) tests, and a discriminant function analysis, using the STEPDISC procedure, and with home versus hospital choice as the classification variable, showed that four of the MATE subscales (inclusion feelings II, control behavior II, control feelings I and II) showed significant univariate effects at $p < .05$, and that the discriminant procedure entered the control feelings I and inclusion behavior II subscales into the classification equation as the best predictors of the nominal variable, with $F(1, 33) = 9.11$, $p < .004$, and $F(1, 33) = 5.59$, $p < .02$, respectively.

DISCUSSION

With regard to the FES, the expressiveness and active/recreational dimensions emerged as important, with families of patients dialyzing at home being seen by patients as relatively more encouraging of direct expression of feelings, though also as somewhat less active in recreational pursuits compared to families of patients dialyzing in hospital.

With regard to partners' responses on the FES, families of patients dialyzing at home, compared to those of patients dialyzing in hospital, were seen as higher in expressiveness, cohesion, and support for independent behavior, and generally lower in need for structure and control.

With regard to the MATE, patients dialyzing at home generally expressed a higher level of intimacy and sensitivity toward the feelings of their partners, while partners of patients dialyzing at home generally showed greater sensitivity toward the patient's need to feel more in control, both in feelings and behavior, and to his or her need to be given more attention.

Analysis of responses to a series of supplementary rating scales completed by both patients and partners showed, in addition, that home patients were generally more satisfied with their treatment procedures and with their choice of dialysis modality than were hospital patients. These data indicated further that the marital relationships of the hospital patients and partners were more likely to be characterized by ambivalence, conflict, uncertainty, and less optimism for future success with the required medical procedures. Similarly, on the MATE, both patients and partners in the hospital dialysis sample showed higher levels of marital relationship dissatisfaction on all subscales than those dialyzing at home, as shown in Tables 1 and 2. There was a higher level of disagreement, or incongruence, between the MATE scores of patients, and those of partners, within the hospital dialysis sample. The rating scale data also showed generally that the extent to which a patient conceived of himself or herself as a "sick patient" was related to dissatisfaction in several aspects of the marital and family situation. There appeared, again, to be marital or family pressure exerted upon patients within the hospital dialysis group to show "appropriate" or correct behavior. By contrast, the home dialysis sample functioned at a higher level in terms of expressiveness, increased activity in political, social, and intellectual concerns, as well as at a generally higher level of overall adjustment both in terms of the family unit itself and of the family's relationship with the dialyzing patient. Both patient and partner satisfaction with their marriage, or other primary relationship, were directly related to greater patient and partner satisfaction with the chosen treatment modality. This type of variable is seldom investigated by renal treatment centers, yet it appears to be important as a source of prognostic data regarding potential adjustment to a major treatment regimen such as dialysis. The FES and MATE data, coupled with that from the supplementary rating scale procedures mentioned above, seem to indicate that the patient choosing hospital dialysis is generally more at risk in terms of psychological, marital, and family variables. Such patients appear more likely to view themselves passively and somewhat dependently; their families generally tend to lack flexibility and expressiveness, and tend to show higher levels of rigidity and control. Such factors, plus the likelihood of somewhat poorer marital adjustment and satisfaction, obviously impede both personal and family adjustment to, and progress with, a dialysis regimen.

It is clear that professionals and others employed in renal treatment centers must be aware of the broader social, marital, and family context in which patients must be treated. Warner (1982) has suggested that psychologists, for example, might well be considered "social systems consultants." In this vein, treatment alternatives and strategies would have maximal opportunity for success when the surrounding marital and family situation is considered in addition to the patient's obvious medical symptomatology. It is critical, however, to be concerned also with the effects of serious treatments, such as dialysis, on one's spouse and on other family members.

Finally, as outlined in Weisberg and Page (in press), economic factors are also relevant. Home dialysis is being increasingly advocated as a cost-saving treatment modality, and Medicare payments for the treatment have been reduced. It is therefore doubly important to study the marital and family context in which such patients must function. Perhaps strategies will have to be developed with the goal of expediting home treatment for patients who might normally choose to undergo the procedures in a hospital. The family and social systems in which these persons must undergo treatment appear to play a considerable role in determining their satisfaction, well-being, and overall progress. An additional area for future research would involve the question of whether social, marital, and family variables with ESRD patients bear some relationship to mortality rates. These types of variables constitute a major area for research in the future, albeit one seldom recognized in the past.

REFERENCES

Beard, B. and T. Sampson. 1981. "Denial and Objectivity in Hemodialysis Patients: Adjustments by Opposite Mechanisms." In N. Levy, ed. *Psychonephrology: Psychosocial Factors in Hemodialysis and Transplantation.* (pp. 300-330). New York: Plenum Press.

Binik, Y. 1983. Coping with Chronic Life-Threatening Illness: Psychosocial Perspectives on End-Stage Renal Disease. *Canadian Journal of Behavioral Science* 15:373-392.

Cummings, J. 1970. "Hemodialysis: Facts, Feelings, and Fantasies." *American Journal of Nursing* 1:70-75.

Drees, A. and E. Gallagher. 1981. "Hemodialysis, Rehabilitation, and Psychological Report." In N. Levy, Ed. *Psychonephrology: Psychological Factors in Hemodialysis and Transplantation* (pp. 210-220). New York: Plenum Press.

Filstead, W. 1979. *Comparing the Family Environments of Alcoholics and Normal Families.* Publication of the Department of Psychiatry and Behavioral Science, Northwestern University.

Friedman, E. 1978. *Strategy in Renal Failure.* New York: Wiley.

Kaplan De-Nour, K. 1981. Prediction of Adjustment to Chronic Hemodialysis. In N. Levy, Ed. *Psychonephrology: Psychological Factors in Hemodialysis and Transplantation* (pp. 35-51). New York: Plenum Press.

Moos, R. and B. Moos. 1981. *Family Environment Scale: Manual.* Palo Alto: Consulting Psychologists Press.

Rasmussen, R. 1980. "Perceived Family Climate and Interpersonal Characteristics of Alcoholic Women and Their Husbands." *Dissertation Abstracts International*, 40, 8-B, 3418.

Schutz, W. 1978. *FIRO Awareness Scales: Manual.* Palo Alto: Consulting Psychologists Press.

Statistical Analysis System Institute. 1985. *Statistical Analysis System (SAS) User's Guide: Statistics.* Cary, NC.

Weisberg, M. 1984. *Personal, Marital, and Family Characteristics of Patients Receiving Dialysis In-center or at Home.* Unpublished doctoral dissertation, University of Windsor.

Weisberg, M. and S. Page. 1988. "The Millon Behavioral Health Inventory and Perceived Efficacy of Home and Hospital Dialysis." *Journal of Social and Clinical Psychology* 8:408-422.

Weisberg, M. and S. Page. (in press). "Personality Variables and Coping with Treatment for Life-Threatening Illness, with Special Reference to Dialysis." In T. Miller, ed. *Chronic Pain: Clinical Readings and Health Care Delivery.* Lexington, KY: International Universities Press.

Warner, R. 1982. "The Psychologist as Social Systems Consultant." In T. Millon, C. Green, and R. Meagher, eds. *Handbook of Clinical Health Psychology* (pp. 45-55). New York: Plenum Press.

Wetzel, J. and F. Raymond. 1980. "A Person-Environment Study of Depression." *Social Service Review* 54:363.

II: PSYCHOSOCIAL DIMENSIONS OF RENAL DISEASE

Psychological and Social Adaptation of CAPD and Center Hemodialysis Patients

Carl A. Maida
Alfred H. Katz
Deane L. Wolcott
John Landsverk
Gayle Strauss
Allen R. Nissenson

Carl A. Maida, PhD, is Assistant Research Anthropologist, Department of Psychiatry and Biobehavioral Sciences, UCLA School of Medicine and School of Public Health. Alfred H. Katz, DSW, is Professor at UCLA School of Public Health and School of Social Welfare, Los Angeles, CA. Deane L. Wolcott, MD, is Assistant Professor, Department of Psychiatry and Biobehavioral Sciences, UCLA School of Medicine, and is Associate Chief, Consultation-Liaison Psychiatry Service, UCLA Neuropsychiatric Institute, Los Angeles, CA. John Landsverk, PhD, is Assistant Research Sociologist, Department of Psychiatry and Biobehavioral Sciences, UCLA School of Medicine. Gayle Strauss, EdD, is Research Assistant, Department of Psychiatry and Biobehavioral Sciences, UCLA School of Medicine, Los Angeles, CA. Allen R. Nissenson, MD, is Associate Professor, Department of Medicine, UCLA School of Medicine, and is Director of the Dialysis Program, UCLA Medical Center, Los Angeles, CA.

The authors wish to express their appreciation to Hector Myers, PhD, of the Department of Psychology, UCLA, Kenneth A. Wallston, PhD, of the Department of Psychology, Vanderbilt University, and Aaron Antonovsky, PhD, of the Department of the Sociology of Health, Ben Gurion University of the Negev, Israel.

Incenter hemodialysis (HD) is the predominant treatment modality for adult dialysis patients in the United States. Continuous ambulatory peritoneal dialysis (CAPD) is an alternative dialytic technique introduced in the late 1970s. Approximately 72,000 individuals with end-stage renal disease (ESRD) were on chronic dialysis in the United State as of the mid-1980s (Freeman 1985). Nearly 9,000 individuals were on CAPD (Steinberg et al. 1985).

Adaptation to chronic illness and its treatment can be conceptualized as a multidimensional process which includes biological, psychological, and social dimensions and their interrelationships (Ware 1984).

ADAPTATION TO CHRONIC HEMODIALYSIS

ESRD and chronic hemodialysis are associated with acute and/or chronic adverse biological effects on almost all organ systems. Neurological and neurobehavioral abnormalities found in ESRD patients on chronic hemodialysis (HD) include peripheral neuropathy (Pierratos et al. 1981), acute and chronic organic mental disorders (Jack, Rabin, and McKinney 1983-84; Stewart and Stewart 1979; Kerr 1980), cognitive performance deficits (Osberg et al. 1982; McKee et al. 1982; Hart et al. 1983; Ryan, Souheaver, and de Wolfe 1981), and electrophysiological function abnormalities (Teschan et al. 1979, 1983).

A high percentage of nondiabetic, and a higher percentage of diabetic, chronic HD patients have physical performance capacity impairment that interferes with personal (self-care, mobility, routine physical activities) as well as vocational function (Gutman, Stead, and Robinson 1981).

In addition, a high incidence of psychological symptoms (anxiety, depression) and of psychiatric syndromes have been documented in chronic HD patients (Baldree, Murphy, and Powers 1982; Stewart 1983; Maher et al. 1983; Livesley 1982; Zetin and Dietch 1983; Kalman, Wilson, and Kalman 1983; Levy 1979).

Finally, chronic HD patients have a high incidence of social function impairment. Family relationship problems include marital conflict, sexual dysfunction, and psychological distress in children of adult HD patients (Blodgett 1981-82; Munakata 1982; Berkman,

Katz, and Weissman 1982; De-Nour 1982; Farmer et al. 1979; Steidl et al. 1980; Levy and Wynbrandt 1975; Conley et al. 1981).

Social and leisure activity restrictions and vocational disability are also ubiquitous in chronic HD patients (Palmer et al. 1983; Johnson, McCauley, and Copley 1982; De-Nour, Shanan, and Garty 1977-78; Kutner and Cardenas 1981; Dc-Nour and Czaczkes 1975).

ADAPTATION TO CAPD

Long-term outcome studies of CAPD and HD indicate that the mortality rate of equivalent patients on these two modalities is similar, but that CAPD patients have a higher rate of hospital days per patient year (Nissenson et al. in press; Nolph, Pyle, and Hialt 1983; Wing et al. 1983; Khanna et al. 1983; Mion et al. 1983). CAPD patients, as compared to HD patients, have adequate biochemical control, higher hematocrits, lower blood pressures, and higher serum triglyceride levels (Levey and Harington 1982) and do not differ in the incidence of osteodystrophy (Freundlich, Zillernelo, and Strauss 1983) or peripheral neuropathy (Pierratos et al. 1981). CAPD has continued to be associated with high rates of infectious complications and treatment drop-out (Steinberg et al. 1985).

Fragola et al. (1983) studied patients from 125 dialysis centers and found that diabetic and nondiabetic CAPD patients had higher Karnovsky scores (indicating higher physical performance capacity) than did comparable groups of HD patients. Further, improved patient psychosocial status, including improved ability to travel, more independence and control over treatment, less treatment-related stress for family members, and improved vocational function, were early advantages for CAPD hoped or claimed by its proponents (Oreopoulos and Khanna 1982; Oreopoulos 1980). However, there is still limited literature on the psychosocial status of CAPD patients. Increased strength and endurance, improved health status, fewer restrictions on fluid intake and diet, decreased modality-related stresses, and increased freedom and ease of travel have been reported. Reported disadvantages have included pain and fear associated with peritonitis, adverse body image effects, the boredom associated with CAPD exchange procedures, and lack of improvement in sexual function and quality of life (Fragola et al. 1983; Geiser et al. 1983-84; Lindsay et al. 1980).

Devins et al. (1983-84) found that CAPD patients did not report their illness/treatment to be less intrusive in nine areas of social, role, and health function than did HD patients. In addition, two previous studies have found that CAPD patients did not have better mood state than HD patients (Lindsay et al. 1980; Devins et al. 1983-84).

No difference in employment rates of CAPD and HD patients was found in one study (Lindsay et al. 1980), and only a slight difference favoring CAPD in this regard when controlling for diabetic status, age, and educational level in another study (Fragola et al. 1983).

Evans et al. (1985) reported on the quality of life of 347 center HD and 81 CAPD patients as part of an 11-center cross-sectional study of all current forms of ESRD treatment. Their CAPD population has a higher percentage of white patients and lower percentage of black patients then did the center HD population. The groups were similar on the variables of age, sex, and mean years of education. Their CAPD population had a lower incidence of hypertensive disease, a higher incidence of diabetic kidney disease, and a lower mean number of comorbid conditions. However, their CAPD patient population, as compared to the center HD population, had slightly more functional impairment (based on Karnovsky scores), a smaller percentage of patients who reported they were able to work (24.7 percent versus 37.2 percent), and they reported marginally higher levels of positive psychological affect, overall life satisfaction, and well-being. Although they controlled statistically for sociodemographic and medical factors, their subjects were drawn from up to 11 centers and they did not report comparative data from each center, leaving open the possibility that patient selection bias and inter-center population mix differences may have confounded their results (Evans et al. 1985).

We undertook the present study to gather further information on the adaptation of CAPD patients as compared to chronic center HD patients. We studied psychological and social status variables cross-scctionally, in matched patient groups, from a single university dialysis program.

The purpose of this approach was to document similarities or dissimilarities in the adaptation of CAPD and center HD patients, and to partially control for patient selection factors that might contribute to any differences in adaptation between these two patient groups.

METHODS

Subject Selection

All center HD and CAPD patients from a university medical center were included in the potential subject pool if they had been on their current treatment modality at least six months, were competent in English, were between the ages of 20 and 65, and had an appropriate match in the other treatment modality. Because of other matching criteria considerations, one patient on CAPD for only three months was included. Exclusionary criteria were chronic psychosis, stroke syndrome or clinical evidence for dementia, major hearing impairment, or major visual impairment (inability to read large print with glasses). The purpose of the exclusionary criteria was to exclude individuals whose level of adaptation would be primarily determined by their nonrenal health status.

Study matching variables were sex, age, interval since chronic dialysis began (independent of modality), presence or absence of diabetes, and ethnicity. These variables were chosen because they may be important determinants of adaptation to ESRD and chronic dialysis (Wallston and Wallston 1981).

The study was explained to potential subjects and written informed consent obtained by one of the study investigators. At the time of this study there were approximately 30 CAPD and 30 center HD patients under treatment at UCLA. They were under the care of the same physician staff, but different nursing staffs. From this larger group of patients 16 matched pairs of subjects actually participated.

STUDY INSTRUMENTS

The demographic questionnaire measured standard demographic characteristics.

Psychological Status Instruments

The psychological status instruments used in this study were the Profile of Mood States (POMS), the Simmons Scale, the Multidimensional Health Locus of Control (MHLOC), the Antonovsky Sense of Coherence (ASOC) Scale, a general disease/treatment stress scale, and a modality-specific disease/treatment stress scale.

The Profile of Mood States (POMS) is a 65-adjective, self-report checklist of frequency of experienced feelings in the previous seven days. The POMS has subscales of tension/anxiety, depression, anger, fatigue, confusion/bewilderment, and vigor. A combined POMS total mood disturbance (TMD) score can also be calculated for each individual. Scoring procedures and reference group norms are available (McNair, Lorr, and Droppleman 1981). The POMS has previously been used in research on medically ill patient groups (Weisman, Worden, and Sobel 1980).

The Simmons Scale is a nine-item measure of self-esteem, adapted from the Rosenberg Self Esteem Scale (Rosenberg 1965) and previously validated and used in Simmons' studies of the psychosocial consequences of kidney transplantation (Simmons, Klein, and Simmons 1977).

The Multidimensional Health Locus of Control (MHLOC) is an 18-item scale composed of three six-item subscales of internality, chance externality, and powerful other dimensions. Extensive reliability and validity testing of the MHLOC has been reported (Wallston and Wallston 1981).

The general disease/treatment stress scale and the modality-specific disease treatment/stress scales were adapted slightly from the scales used by Lindsay and Burton in their study of adaptation of CAPD and home HD patients in Ontario (Wai et al. 1981).

The Antonovsky Sense of Coherence Scale is a 35-item scale that assesses subjects' understanding and reactions to their illness along the dimensions of comprehensibility, manageability, meaningfulness, and a global sense of illness understanding (coherence) (Antonovsky 1983, 1984).

Cognitive performance and electrophysiological function were also assessed in these patients. The protocols used and the results will be reported in other papers.

Social Status Instruments

Several measures of social and role function were used. Brief scales assessed subjects' perceptions of the stresses their family members and friends had experienced due to patient illness and treatment in the previous three months. Subjects' perceptions of the quality of their current relationships with their dialysis physicians(s), dialysis nurses, and other dialysis patients were assessed by self-report. Current vocational function was assessed by use of an author-constructed Vocational Status Questionnaire.

Social support and social network characteristics and family interactional patterns were also assessed in these patients. The Myers Resources and Social Supports Measures (RSSM) assessed seven key variables: (1) the number of important persons in the support network, (2) the pattern of relationships within the network, (3) the multidimensionality of the network, (4) the relative importance of five types of support received, (5) the degree of satisfaction with the support received in each of these areas, (6) the density of the social network, and (7) reciprocity within the social network.

The Family Environment Scale (FES) assesses the social environment of families along ten salient dimensions. It focuses on the measurement and description of the interpersonal relationships among family members, on the directions of personal growth emphasized within the family, and on the basic organizational structure of the family.

Data Collection

Because of the number of study instruments and the complexity of this study, data collection was divided into four separate blocks: electrophysiological measures, neuropsychological tests, and two psychosocial test points. The total testing time required for these four data collection points was about 4-1/2 hours. Most of the data were collected from the HD subjects within 7-14 days, as almost all of the "psychosocial" data could be obtained while the patient was on dialysis. The collection of the data on CAPD patients usually occurred over a longer time interval, as these patients usually attended clinic only once every six weeks.

Data Reduction and Analysis

Data on the matching and other demographic variables was grouped according to treatment modality.

Psychological Status Variables

The POMS, Simmons, MHLOC, and Antonovsky Sense of Coherence Scales were scored according to standardized criteria. Higher POMS subscale and "Total Mood Disturbance" scores indicate increased emotional distress in the preceding seven days. The potential range of Simmons' Scale scores is 0-9, with higher scores indicating more self-esteem. Higher scores on the three MHLOC subscales indicate the attribution of more control over illness outcome to "internal," "powerful others," and "chance external" forces. Higher ASOC subscale scores indicate the subjects have a stronger perception of the meaningfulness, comprehensibility, and manageability of their illness and its treatment.

The "general disease/treatment stress" score was summed from individuals' responses to 16 questions concerning "modality-independent," illness-related physiological and psychological stresses. The "modality-specific disease/treatment stress" score was summed from individuals' responses to 11 questions about specific stresses related to HD or CAPD. Different items were used for the modality-specific disease/treatment stress questionnaire for each subject group, and the HD and CAPD group scores are not necessarily comparable on this scale.

Social Status Variables

The FES (Moos 1981) and Myers Resources and Social Supports Measure (Myers 1981) were scored according to standardized criteria. The "Illness-Related Social Network Stress" responses were dichotomized into reports of very much/extreme, versus lesser degree of, stress on social network members in the previous three months. The "Relationship Quality" responses were dichotomized into very good/excellent versus less good current relationship quality.

After scoring of each of the instruments and scales, Pearson product-moment correlations of the continuous sociodemographic, psychological, and social variable scores were calculated. Group differences were assessed by means of paired "T" tests.

RESULTS

Table 1 shows the results of the study matching variables for the CAPD and CHD groups, as well as comparisons of their educational history and marital status. On the study matching variables, the two groups were very closely matched, with the important exception that the HD group had more patients with underlying diabetes.

Table 2 shows the results of social support and family interactional variables. The two groups were very similar in social network, size, dimensionality, density, and reciprocity. There were statistically significant group differences in the pattern of relationships. The CAPD group self-reported more supportive ties outside the family and the network of health providers. The HD group attached greater importance to the advice received from those in their networks. The two groups were quite comparable in family interactional patterns. The HD group, however, scored higher on the Achievement Orientation subscale of the FES. The mean scores for the study population on the FES were compared to those of a group of normal families (N = 1125) (Moos 1981). The CAPD group scored equally to, or higher than, the normal families on eight of the ten dimensions, the exceptions being Conflict and Control. The HD group scored higher than the normal families on six dimensions, and only slightly below the norms in Conflict, Intellectual/Cultural Orientation, Active-Recreational Orientation, and Control.

Figure 1 shows the group mean POMS subscale and total mood disturbance (TMD) scores for the CAPD and HD subjects with reference to norms from a previously assessed health college student group (N = 856) (McNair, Lorr, and Droppleman 1981). Although

TABLE 1. Matching and Sociodemographic Characteristics of CAPD and Center HD Patients

CHARACTERISTIC	CAPD (N=16)	CENTER HD (N=16)
SEX (% of patients)		
Male	68.8	68.8
Female	31.2	31.2
AGE (mean years)	41.0	42.6
RACE/ETHNICITY (% of patients)		
Caucasian	56.2	43.8
Black	31.2	31.2
Asian American	12.5	6.2
Hispanic	0.0	12.5
American Indian	0.0	6.2
MARITAL STATUS		
Never Married	56.2	37.5
Married	43.8	43.8
Divorced/Widowed	0.0	18.7
EDUCATION (mean years)	14.6	14.8
DIABETES (% of patients)	6.2	18.8
TIME SINCE ONSET ANY DIALYSIS		
Mean (months)	73.2	70.1
Range (months)	3 to 204	7 to 178

the group mean scores for the CAPD subjects were lower on each of the five negative mood POMS subscales, and for the combined POMS-TMD score (indicating less current emotional distress in the CAPD group), these differences did not reach statistical significance, perhaps due to sample size. The mean POMS subscale scores of both groups were well within one standard deviation of the group mean scores of the college student reference group on all six subscales.

Table 3 shows the results of other study measures of psychological well-being/distress in the two subject groups. There were no statistically significant group differences in self-esteem (Simmons' scale), on the three subscales of the Multidimensional Health Locus

TABLE 2. Measures of Social Support for CAPD and Center HD Patients

MEASURE	CAPD (N=16)	CENTER HD (N=16)
MYERS RESOURCES AND SOCIAL SUPPORT MEASURE (means)		
# Available Supports	11.0	12.0
Pattern of Relations		
Spouse	0.4	0.6
Nuclear Family	3.2	3.0
Relative	0.9	1.0
In-Law	0.4	0.4
Medical	0.2	0.5
All Other	2.2	1.0 *
Multidimensionality		
1 Activity	3.6	3.5
1+ Activity	7.6	8.6
Index of Multidimensionality	0.7	0.6
Importance of Support		
Advice	28.3	39.7 *
Praise/Criticism	32.3	39.6
Socializing	36.6	44.0
Specific Help	36.2	39.4
Emotional Support	37.1	42.3
Satisfaction with Support		
Advice	11.5	14.1
Praise/Criticism	11.2	13.6
Socializing	13.2	12.6
Specific Help	15.0	14.4
Emotional Support	14.9	16.8
Network Density		
Relatives	36.1	36.5
Friends	24.0	13.6
Others	8.4	4.4
Overall Density	5.4	4.0
Reciprocity	0.8	0.7
FAMILY ENVIRONMENT SCALE[1] (means)		
Cohesion	7.9	7.4
Expressiveness	6.3	5.6
Conflict	2.7	2.9
Independence	7.1	7.1
Achievement Orientation	5.0	6.6 *
Intellectual/Cultural Orientation	6.5	5.3
Active/Recreational Orientation	5.1	4.2
Moral/Religious Emphasis	5.3	5.3
Organization	6.1	6.4
Control	3.6	4.0

[1] CAPD N=14, Center HD N=14

* p$\leq$ .05

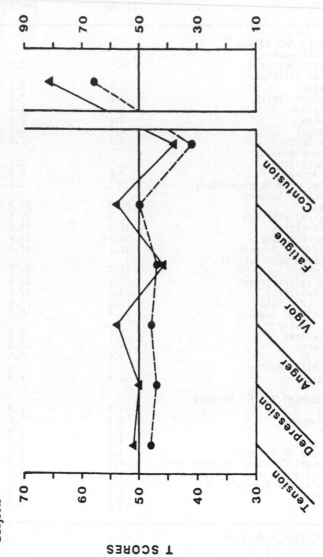

FIGURE 1. Group POMS Subscale and Total Mood Disturbance (TMD) Scores of CAPD and Center HD Subjects

TMD RAW SCORES

T SCORES

● CAPD subjects (N=16)
▲ Center HD subjects (N=16)

Tension Depression Anger Vigor Fatigue Confusion

TABLE 3. Measures of Psychological Well-Being for CAPD and Center HD
Patients

MEASURE	CAPD (N=16)	CENTER HD (N=16)	
SELF-ESTEEM — SIMMONS (mean)	5.0	5.1	
MULTIDIMENSIONAL HEALTH LOCUS OF CONTROL (means)			
Internal	27.2	24.3	
Chance Externa	18.3	17.4	
Powerful Others	25.9	22.6	
ANTONOVSKY SENSE OF COHERENCE (means)			
Comprehensibility	20.2	19.9	
Manageability	18.9	20.1	
Meaningfulness	16.6	16.9	
Sense of Coherence	55.8	56.9	
DISEASE/TREATMENT STRESSES			
General (G)	29.1	34.3	
Modality Specific (MS)	21.3	18.9	
Total (G + MS)	50.4	53.2	
DISEASE/TREATMENT RELATED STRESSES (% of patients reporting very or extremely stressful — last three months)			
Low Energy/Easily exhausted	18.8	56.2	**
Trouble Sleeping	0.0	31.2	**
High Blood Pressure	6.7	12.5	
Headache	0.0	12.5	
Trouble Concentrating	13.3	18.8	
Decreased Appetite	13.3	37.5	
Bone Pain	0.0	25.0	**
Loss of Sensation	0.0	18.8	*
Muscle Weakness	20.0	50.0	*
Shortness of Breath	20.0	31.2	
Fluid Restriction	6.7	50.0	***
Diet Restrictions	13.3	68.8	***
Itching	0.0	12.5	
Difficulty Traveling Because of TX	20.0	50.0	*
Medical Tests/Procedures	13.3	31.2	
Hospitalization	6.7	37.5	**

*   p< .10
**   p< .05
*** p< .01

of Control (MHLOC), on the three subscales and the global "coherence" scores of the Antonovsky Sense of Coherence Scale, or on the general disease/treatment stress or modality-specific stress scale scores. However the CAPD group consistently, and often significantly, reported less distress from common physical symptoms or treatment restrictions.

The CAPD patient group had slightly higher "internal" and "powerful other" scores on the MHLOC. Higher "internal" locus of control has been associated with better treatment compliance and treatment outcome in previous studies of HD patients (Munakata 1982; De-Nour, Shanan, and Garty 1977-78; Wenerowicz, Riskind, and Jenkins 1978; Zetin et al. 1981; Poll and De-Nour 1980; Viederman 1978; Goldstein 1976; Parker 1983).

Table 4 shows the study results of the social/role function variables. A significantly smaller percentage of CAPD than HD patients reported a high degree of illness/treatment related stresses on members on their social network. A higher percentage of CAPD patients reported very good/excellent relationships with dialysis physicians, nurses, and other patients.

More CAPD as compared to HD subjects reported their current employment status as full-time work/student, and fewer described themselves as unemployed.

Intercorrelations of the Study Variables

The POMS-TMD, Simmons' Scale, and four ASOC subscales were highly, and usually significantly, intercorrelated for the dialysis subjects as a whole, and for the CAPD and center HD subgroups. The three MHLOC subscales were not correlated with the POMS-TMD, ASOC subscales, general disease/treatment stress, or modality-specific disease/treatment stress scores for the subject groups. The MHLOC "internal" and "chance" subscale scores were nonsignificantly correlated with the Simmons' Scale scores in the CAPD group. The MHLOC "internal" and "powerful others" subscale scores were highly significantly correlated (p ≤ .01) with the index of multidimensionality on the Myers RSSM. The MHLOC "chance" subscale score was usually significantly correlated (p ≤ .05) with the FES "organization" dimension. The four

TABLE 4. Measures of Social Activity and Relationships for CAPD and Center Patients

MEASURES	CAPD (N=16)	CENTER HD (N=16)
ILLNESS RELATED STRESS ON (% patients reporting very much or extreme)		
Self	13.3	37.5 ***
Spouse/Partner 1	0.0	66.7 ***
Other Family 2	16.7	37.5
Closest Friend 3	16.7	37.5 ***
TOTAL ILLNESS SOCIAL NETWORK STRESS (% of patients reporting very much or extreme stress for at least one network member)	12.5	43.8 ***
QUALITY OF RELATIONSHIP (% of patients reporting very good or excellent)		
Dialysis Physicians	80.0	43.8 **
Dialysis Nurses	93.3	68.8 *
Other Dialysis Patients	83.3	18.8 ***
EMPLOYMENT STATUS (% of patients)		
Full-Time Work/Study	37.5	18.7
Part-Time Work/Study	12.5	12.5
Housewife	6.2	6.2
Unemployed	43.8	62.6

*   p< .10
**   p< .05
*** p< .01

1. CAPD N=7, Center HD N=9
2. CAPD N=6, Center HD N=8
3. CAPD N=12, Center HD N=16

ASOC subscales were highly and usually significantly intercorrelated with the Myers RSSM. The key subscale, "coherence," was highly significantly correlated with the density of relatives on the RSSM, and usually significantly correlated with the number of supports and the advice, socializing and emotional support that subjects received from their social networks. The FES "conflict" dimension was highly significantly correlated with the number of supports, density of relatives, and the overall average density of the subjects' social networks. The FES "achievement orientation" dimension was highly significantly correlated with the advice and specific help that subjects received from their networks. The FES "independence" dimension was highly significantly correlated, negatively, with the density of friends and the overall average density of the social network. The FES "expressiveness" dimension was usually significantly correlated with reciprocity within the social network. The FES and the Myers RSSM were not correlated with the POMS-TMD.

The general and modality-specific disease/treatment stress scores showed no consistent pattern of correlations with the time in months since dialysis onset, subject age, or any of the other psychological well-being variables.

Except for diabetic status, the subjects in the CAPD and HD groups were quite comparable with respect to the study matching and other sociodemographic variables. This study did not assess physical performance capacity, which may or may not significantly differ in appropriately matched CAPD and center HD patient groups (Evans et al. 1985).

Both CAPD and center HD subject groups showed only moderate differences from normal or healthy historical reference groups on the POMS, MHLOC, FES, Simmons' Scale, and ASOC. Thus their psychological adaptations appear to be remarkably well preserved and positive. The CAPD subjects' trend to lower POMS scores and lower general disease/treatment stress cores, and their pattern of reporting less distress from physical symptoms and treatment restrictions, is consistent with findings from most previous literature that CAPD is associated with lesser psychological distress (Fragola et al. 1983; Geiser et al. 1983-84; Lindsay et al. 1980; Evans et al. 1985). Results of the measures of cognitive function, as assessed by neuropsychological testing and electrophysiological function, were consistently better or more "normal" in CAPD subjects.

The CAPD patients also indicated fewer problems in their general social adaptation; they reported less disease/treatment stress on members of their intimate social network, a higher rate of structured vocational activities, and better relationships with dialysis physicians, nurses, and other dialysis patients. Thus there is a consistent trend in our results indicating that, in medically comparable CAPD and center HD patients, the psychological and social dimensions of adaptation of CAPD patients are marginally to moderately superior.

DISCUSSION

Potential limitations on the reliability and generalizability of this study include the small sample size, the fact that these subjects were patients at an academic medical dialysis program, and some special sample characteristics (e.g., the long mean duration of dialysis for both groups). The study has been extended to another dialysis center to see if the findings generalize across institutional boundaries, and to enlarge the sample size.

Our findings do not provide support to the proposition that CAPD patients have *significantly superior* adaptation in comparison to medically and sociodemographically similar center HD patients. It is possible that there are consistent baseline psychosocial differences between patients who select center HD as compared to CAPD, which may confound true modality-related effects on patient adaptation.

Although conclusions cannot be drawn from this study about modality preferences, the data do suggest that center HD patients who experience significant chronic distress from marked fatigue, weakness, sleep disorder, and restrictions on diet, fluid, and travel, and those who find their treatment to be very stressful for members of their social network, might find these problems less severe if they changed to CAPD. However, we do not currently know if reporting of distress in these areas is a modality-related or personality-related characteristic. Current evidence is not strong that CAPD is associated with superior physical performance capacity as measured by medical observer-rated Karnovsky scores. The evidence is mixed as to whether CAPD is associated with improved or poorer vocational status, as compared to center hemodialysis patients.

A major task of research on differential adaptation to CAPD and HD is to identify profiles of individuals who can be predicted to achieve a higher level of adaptation on one of the available ESRD treatment modalities. Such a profile would then be useful to physicians and patients as they make modality selection choices. Another goal of such research would be to identify those individuals at high risk for treatment noncompliance, modality dropout, or poor adaptation on a given modality, and to determine which psychosocial interventions are efficacious in preventing these adverse outcomes.

Prospective longitudinal studies are needed which multidimensionally assess the adaptation of patients prior to the onset of dialysis, and which follow those who elect a given dialysis modality over time, so that pretreatment levels of adaptation, and both modality-nonspecific and modality-specific dialysis consequences, can be successfully discriminated.

Given the size and costs of the ESRD program, the economic factors in treatment-modality selection, the high current CAPD drop-out rate for patient choice, and treatment noncompliance (Evans et al. 1985), such longitudinal studies should have a high priority.

REFERENCES

Antonovsky, A. 1983. "The Sense of Coherence: Development of a Research Instrument." Newsletter and research reports, William S. Schwartz Research Center for Behavioral Medicine, Tel-Aviv University, Israel.

Antonovsky, A. 1984. "The Sense of Coherence as a Determinant of Health." In J. D. Matarazzo, J. A. Herd, N. E. Miller, and S. M. Weiss, eds. *Behavioral Health*. New York: J. Wiley, pp. 114-129.

Baldree, K. S., S. P. Murphy, and M. J. Powers. 1982. "Stress Identification and Coping Patterns in Patients on Hemodialysis." *Nursing Research* 31:107-112.

Berkman, A. H., L. A. Katz, and R. Weissman. 1982. "Sexuality and the Life-Style of Home Dialysis Patients." *Archives of Physical and Medical Rehabilitation* 63:272-275.

Blodgett, C. 1981-1982. "A Selected Review of the Literature of Adjustment to Hemodialysis." *International Journal of Psychiatric Medicine* 11:97-124.

Conley, J. A., H. J. Burton, A. K. De-Nour, and G. A. Wells. 1981. "Support Systems for Patients and Spouses on Home Dialysis." *International Journal of Family Psychiatry* 2:45-54.

De-Nour, A. K. 1982. "Social Adjustment of Chronic Dialysis Patients." *American Journal of Psychiatry* 139:97-100.

De-Nour, A. K. and J. W. Czaczkes. 1975. "Personality Factors Influencing Vocational Rehabilitation." *Archives of General Psychiatry* 32:573-577.

De-Nour, A. K., J. Shanan, and I. Garty. 1977-78. "Coping Behavior and Intelligence in the Prediction of Vocational Rehabilitation of Dialysis Patients." *International Journal of Psychiatric Medicine* 8:145-158.

Devins, G. M., Y. M. Binik, T. A., Hutchinson et al. 1983-1984. "The Emotional Impact of End-Stage Renal Disease: Importance of Patients' Perceptions of Intrusiveness and Control." *International Journal of Psychiatric Medicine* 13:327-343.

Evans, R. W., D. L. Manninen, L. P. Garrison, Jr., L. G. Hart, C. R. Blagg, R. A. Gutman, A. R. Hall, and E. G. Lowrie. 1985. *New England Journal of Medicine* 312:553-559.

Farmer, C. J., M. Bewick, V. Parsons, and S. A. Snowden. 1979. "Survival on Home Haemodialysis: Its Relationship with Physical Symptomatology, Psychosocial Background and Psychiatric Morbidity." *Psychological Medicine* 9:515-523.

Fragola, J. A., S. Grube, L. Von Bloch, and E. Bourke. 1983. "Multicentre Study of Physical Activity and Employment Status of Continuous Ambulatory Peritoneal Dialysis (CAPD) Patients in the United States." *Proceedings of the EDTA* 20:243-249.

Freeman, R. B. 1985. "Treatment of Chronic Renal Failure: An Update." *New England Journal of Medicine* 312:577-579.

Freundlich, M., G. Zillernelo, and J. Strauss. 1983. "Mineral Metabolism in Children and Adults Receiving Continuous Ambulatory Peritoneal Dialysis." *Seminal Nephrology* 3:159-163.

Geiser, M. T., C. Van Dyke, R. East, and M. Weiner, 1983-84. "Psychological Reactions to Continuous Ambulatory Peritoneal Dialysis." *International Journal of Psychiatric Medicine* 13:299-307.

Goldstein, A. M. 1976. "Denial and External Locus of Control as Mechanisms of Adjustment in Chronic Medical Illness." *Essence* 1:5-22.

Gutman, R. A., W. W. Stead, and R. R. Robinson. 1981. "Physical Activity and Employment Status of Patients on Maintenance Dialysis." *New England Journal of Medicine* 304:309-313.

Hart, R. P., J. A. Pederson, A. W. Czerwinskil, and R. L. Adams. 1983. "Chronic Renal Failure, Dialysis, and Neuropsychological Function." *Journal of Clinical Neuropsychology* 5:301-312.

Jack, R., P. L. Rabin, and T. D. McKinney. 1983-84. "Dialysis Encephalopathy: A Review." *International Journal of Psychiatric Medicine* 13:309-325.

Johnson, J. P., C. R. McCauley, and J. B. Copley. 1982. "The Quality of Life of Hemodialysis and Transplant Patients." *Kidney International* 22:286-291.

Kalman, T. P., P. G. Wilson, and C. M. Kalman. 1983. "Psychiatric Morbidity in Long Term Renal Transplant Recipients and Patients Undergoing Hemodialysis: A Comparative Study." *Journal of the American Medical Association* 250:55-58.

Kerr, D. N. S. 1980. "Clinical and Pathophysiologic Changes in Patients on Chronic Dialysis: The Central Nervous System." *Advances in Nephrology* 9:109-132.

Khanna, R., G. Wu, S. Vas, and D. G. Oreopoulos. 1983. "Mortality and Morbidity on CAPD." *ASAIO Journal* 6:197-204.

Kutner, N. G. and D. D. Cardenas. 1981. "Rehabilitation Status of Chronic Renal Disease Patients Undergoing Dialysis: Variations by Age Category." *Archives of Physical and Medical Rehabilitation* 62:626-630.

Levey, A. S. and J. T. Harington. 1982. "Continuous Peritoneal Dialysis for Chronic Renal Failure." *Medicine* (Baltimore) 61:330-339.

Levy, N. B. 1979. "Psychological Problems of the Patient on Hemodialysis and Their Treatment." *Psychotherapy Psychosomatic* 31:235-242.

Levy, N. B. and G. D. Wynbrandt. 1975. "The Quality of Life on Maintenance Hemodialysis." *Lancet* 1(7920):1328-1330.

Lindsay, R. M., D. G. Oreopoulos, H. Burton et al. 1980. "Adaptation to Home Dialysis: A Comparison of Continuous Ambulatory Peritoneal Dialysis and Hemodialysis." *Proceedings of the First International Symposium on CAPD, Amsterdam, Excerpta Medica*, pp. 120-130.

Livesley, W. J. 1982. "Symptoms of Anxiety and Depression in Patients Undergoing Chronic Hemodialysis." *Journal of Psychosomatic Research* 26:581-584.

Maher, B. A., D. L. Lamping, C. A. Dickinson et al. 1983. "Psychosocial Aspects of Chronic Hemodialysis: The National Cooperative Dialysis Study." *Kidney International* (Supplement 13) 23:S-50-57.

McKee, D. C., G. B. Burnett, D. D. Raft et al. 1982. "Longitudinal Study of Neuropsychological Functioning in Patients on Chronic Hemodialysis: A Preliminary Report." *Journal of Psychosomatic Research* 26:511-518.

McNair, D. M., M. Lorr, and L. F. Droppleman. 1981. *Manual for the Profile of Mood States*. San Diego, CA: Educational and Industrial Testing Service.

Mion, C. M., G. Mourad, B. Canand et al. 1983. "Maintenance Dialysis: A Summary of 17 Years Experience in Langeudoc-Rousillon with a Comparison of Methods in a Standard Population." *ASAIO Journal* 6:205-213.

Moos, R. H. 1981. *Manual for the Family Environment Scale (FES)*. Palo Alto, CA: Consulting Psychologists Press.

Munakata, T. 1982. "Psychosocial Influence on Self-care of the Hemodialysis Patient." *Social Science Medicine* 16:1253-1264.

Myers, H. 1981. Resources and social supports measure. Department of Psychology, University of California, Los Angeles and Department of Psychiatry and Human Behavior, Charles R. Drew Medical School, Los Angeles.

Nissenson, A. R., D. E. Gentile, R. E. Soderblom, and C. Brax. (In press). "Medical Review Board, NCC No. 4: Morbidity and Mortality of CAPD-Regional Experience and Long-term Prospects." *American Journal of Kidney Disease*.

Nolph, K. D., W. K. Pyle, and M. Hialt. 1983. "Mortality and Morbidity in CAPD." *ASAIO Journal* 6:220-226.

Oreopoulos, D. G. 1980. "An Update on Continuous Ambulatory Peritoneal Dialysis (CAPD)." *International Journal of Artificial Organs* 3:231-234.

Oreopoulos, D. G. and R. Khanna. 1982. "The Present and Future Role of Continuous Ambulatory Peritoneal Dialysis (CAPD)." *American Journal of Kidney Disease* 2:381-385.

Osberg, J. W., G. J. Meares, D. C. McKee, and G. B. Burnett. 1982. "Intellectual Functioning in Renal Failure and Chronic Dialysis." *Journal of Chronic Diseases* 35:445-457.

Palmer, S., L. Canzona, J. Conley, and G. Wells. 1983. "Vocational Adaptation of Patients on Home Dialysis: Its Relationship to Personality, Activities and Support Received." *Journal of Psychosomatic Research* 27:201-207.

Parker, J. 1983. "Health Locus of Control: Implications for an End-Stage Renal Disease Program." *AAANNT Journal* 10:29-35.

Pierratos, A., R. D. G. Blain, R. Khanna, C. Quinton, and D. G. Oreopoulos. 1981. "Nerve Electrophysiological Parameters in Patients Undergoing CAPD over Two Years." In G. M. Gohl, M. Kessel, and K. D. Nolph, eds. *Advances in Peritoneal Dialysis*. Oxford: Excerpta Medica Publishers, pp. 341-346.

Poll, B. and A. K. De-Nour. 1980. "Locus of Control and Adjustment to Chronic Haemodialysis." *Psychological Medicine* 10:153-157.

Rosenberg, M. 1965. *Society and the Adolescent Self-Image*. Princeton, NJ: Princeton University Press.

Ryan, J. J., G. T. Souheaver, and A. S. de Wolfe. 1981. "Halstead-Reitan Test Results in Chronic Hemodialysis." *Journal of Nervous and Mental Disease* 169:311-314.

Simmons, R. G., S. D. Klein, and R. L. Simmons. 1977. "Gift of Life: The Social and Psychological Impact of Organ Transplantation." New York: John Wiley, 1977.

Steidl, J. H., O. F. Finkelstein, J. P. Wexler et al. 1980. "Medical Condition, Adherence to Treatment Regimens, and Family Functioning: Their Interactions in Patients Receiving Long-term Dialysis Treatment." *Archives of General Psychiatry* 37:1025-1027.

Steinberg, S. M., S. J. Cutler, J. W. Novak, and K. D. Nolph. 1985. *Report of the National CAPD Registry*. National Institutes of Health, January.

Stewart, R. S. 1983. "Psychiatric Issues in Renal Dialysis and Transplantation." *Hospital Community Psychiatry* 34:623-628.

Stewart, R. S. and Stewart, R. M. 1979. "Neuropsychiatric Aspects of Chronic Renal Disease. *Psychosomatics* 20:524-531.

Teschan, P. E., H. E. Ginn, J. E. Bourne et al. 1979. "Quantitative Indices of Clinical Uremia." *Kidney International* 15:676-697.

Teschan, P. E., H. E. Ginn, R. B. Reed, and J. W. Ward. 1983. "Electrophysiological and Neurobehavioral Responses to Therapy: The National Cooperative Dialysis Study." *Kidney International* 23 (Supplement 13):S-58-65.

Viederman, M. 1978. "On the Vicissitudes of the Need for Control in Patients Confronted with Hemodialysis." *Comprehensive Psychiatry* 19:455-467.

Wai, L., J. Richmond, H. Burton, and R. M. Lindsay. 1981. "Influence of Psychosocial Factors on Survival of Home Dialysis Patient." *Lancet* 2:1155-1156.

Wallston, K. A. and B. S. Wallston. 1981. "Health Locus of Control Scales." In H. M. Lefcourt, ed. *Research with the Locus of Control Construct. Vol. 1: Assessment Methods.* New York: Academic, pp. 189-243.

Ware, J. E. 1984. "Conceptualizing Disease Impact and Treatment Outcomes." *Cancer* 53:2316-2323.

Weisman, A. D., J. W. Worden, and H. J. Sobel. 1980. *Psychosocial Screening and Intervention with Cancer Patients.* National Cancer Institute publication CA#19797.

Wenerowicz, W. J., J. H. Riskind, and P. G. Jenkins. 1978. "Locus of Control and Degree of Compliance in Hemodialysis Patients." *Journal of Dialysis* 2:495-505.

Wing, A. J., M. Broyer, F. P. Brunner et al. 1983. "The Contribution of CAPD in Europe." *ASAIO Journal* 6:214-219.

Zetin, M. and J. Dietch. 1983. "Diagnosing and Treating the Depressed Hemodialysis Patient." *International Journal of Artificial Organs* 6:109-112.

Zetin, M., M. J. Plummer, N. S. Vaziri, and M. Cramer. 1981. "Locus of Control and Adjustment to Chronic Hemodialysis." *Clinical Experience in Dialytic Apheresis* 5:319-334.

Artificial Organs, Organ Transplantation, and Dealing with Death

Allen P. Fertziger

The ability to surgically replace a nonfunctional or dying organ with one from a donor may be among the foremost technological accomplishments of modern medical science. Owing to the highly complex nature of this process, the natural tendency of most physicians has been to focus almost all of their attention on the physical aspects of organ transplants and relatively little on the psychological dimensions. This discussion examines several of these psychological dimensions and pays special attention to key thanatological themes: loss, grief, and dealing with death.

THE PARADOX OF POST-TRANSPLANT DEPRESSION AND NONCOMPLIANCE

Because a successful organ transplant is clearly a cause of celebration both by patient and provider, it often comes as a surprise to discover unexpected psychological problems that follow transplant success. Psychological depression appears to take hold of many recipients, while a number fail to take prescribed immunosuppressant medication that is so critical for preventing tissue rejection. Why do recipients of life-sustaining organs find themselves in the throes of a clinical depression? Why would patients who have longed for a replacement organ, often for major periods of their lives, suddenly engage in such self-destructive behavior? Though questions like these continue to perplex clinicians who manage the postoperative

Allen P. Fertziger, PhD, is an independent scholar in Chevy Chase, MD.

treatment of organ transplant recipients, their regularity has now made psychiatric liaison an almost routine practice in the postoperative strategy. Let us try to create a context that will enable us to understand this unexpected, seemingly paradoxical behavior.

TRANSPLANTATION AND THE ISSUE(S) OF DEATH

Throughout the development of transplant technology, the primary aim, understandably enough, has been on developing successful means to effect mechanical replacement for nonfunctional organs. The logic of organ transplantation has been almost exclusively a logic of mechanical exchange—not unlike the way we "replace" individual components in our automobiles—and the brilliant technology that now accompanies the transplantation process has evolved to surgically effect the exchange and to keep the replacement "body part" alive and well in the recipient's body. Probably because this logic is so fundamentally similar to the kind we routinely apply to many of our machines, we have tended to overlook the human or psychological issues, ones that constitute the core of thanatological thought.

Transplantation of body parts is only analogous to replacing machine parts; there are numerous human complications that finally limit the value of analogy and even falsify it. (To say body part suggests the mechanical, while organ suggests organism—that which is alive.) To begin with, the organ is placed in a living, conscious human being who has hopes, fears, and undoubtedly many other emotions of which we know little. While physicians who treat a patient with a failing or minimally functional organ are primarily concerned with establishing a functional organ replacement capable of supporting life, the patient must also contend with the fear (and reality) that his or her physical body is literally dying. That consciousness or awareness of death, be it the "death" of a single individual organ part like a kidney or the death of the entire body—is, in fact, the central issue in thanatology. Once we enter into this awareness of death, life takes on a wholly different quality, and the intervention of thanatological thought and practice has proven to be a powerful therapeutic force. However, before considering thanatological interventions that may be appropriate to the transplant patient, let us first examine how this awareness of death can complicate the life of the transplant candidate and the successful transplant recipient.

If a patient is considering or being considered for a transplant then we can be certain the potential recipient is a victim of a failing or nonfunctional organ. Though the physician's general response may be to provide some form of therapeutic replacement, either through drugs or surgical replacement, to the patient this event must at some level be experienced as a personal death. Like the death of a loved one in our youth, this personal encounter with death is far less traumatic and debilitating than our own death, but it is nonetheless a death and will have to be grieved. The demise of a once functional and healthy organ that accompanies every transplanted organ is also one of a series of progressive encounters with the ultimate human vulnerability that death represents. Just as our progressive encounters with old age slowly make us aware that we are nearing our death, the encounter with the decision to replace a dying organ does this in an accelerated way.

And if the more symbolic encounter with a dying organ isn't enough to force the transplant candidate into the arena of death and dying, the fact that transplant surgery is invariably a last-ditch life-saving strategy is surely enough to ensure a very striking awareness of personal death. So despite the fact that organ transplant candidates are often openly embraced by strong social supports and widespread community optimism and encouragement, their inner world is highly susceptible to assault by the awareness of death.

MANAGING THE GRIEF
OF THE TRANSPLANT PATIENT

To the thanatologist, the awareness of death constitutes what is probably the primary symptom around which all other interventions are addressed. Clearly, for the terminally ill and/or those who are grieving the loss of a close loved one, this awareness expresses itself in what is known in the thanatological literature as the stages of the process known as grief. This process invariably begins with some sort of shock response when death suddenly forces its inevitable presence into awareness. To the degree that we are psychologically prepared to handle this experience, we either categorically deny the possibility of death, at one end of the grief spectrum, or accept it and move on with productive living, at the other.

Since the primary "dis-ease" seen by thanatologists usually involves something as abstract and ill-defined as conscious awareness, it is often very difficult to pinpoint the source of suffering or dis-ease. When there is a clearly defined loss, the task is much more easy and obvious; however, when the loss itself is abstract, it is often very difficult to connect the cause of suffering with the symptoms of grief. The situation in which a patient with a failing organ is to receive a healthy donor organ is one such case where it is difficult to pinpoint grief. The medical teams performing the transplant procedure are prepared for successful and healthy replacement. When that possibility becomes a reality, there is an understandable cause for celebration and not the slightest reason to grieve.

Like any generic change or transformation from an old "form" to a new "form," there is an obligation for the old (i.e., what is being replaced) *to die* and for the new replacement to be born. However, it is far more natural to celebrate a reborn or newly transplanted organ than it is to grieve the loss of the discarded original, which once was part of the working integrity of the transplant patient. It is this propensity to celebrate the one and deny the other that may be contributing to some of the unexpected and/or paradoxical behaviors that are showing up in otherwise successful transplant procedures.

Stated in another way, I would suggest that failure of successful transplant patients to grieve the loss of their transplanted organ and to express the natural awareness of death that their conditions have created, may be expressing itself in a number of pathological or self-destructive ways. Everyone around them (especially their physicians) has expected them to be ecstatic: they, however, may be experiencing a sense of loss or closeness to death that must be expressed. I further suggest that because of the tendency by physicians and family to overlook the inevitable loss that every transplant creates, the recipient has felt his or her grief to be largely unsanctioned. Almost like the bride or groom whose sense of loss and sadness (from many things including losing their singularity) is often obscured by everyone else's joy and celebration, the transplant recipients probably see themselves as crazy for experiencing a sadness when they know they should be happy.

This type of unsanctioned grief can wreak havoc with transplant recipients who become psychologically victimized; they know they should be happy, but are tugged in another direction by their unsanctioned (and often unexpressed) grief. They have almost no other way to understand or explain such bizarre feelings than to conclude that they must be crazy or weird. When the psychological pressure created by this type of inner chaos is added to the psychological stress of adjusting to a fairly radical change in life-style, the combination can be more than the transplant patient can handle.

For these reasons, it is essential that clinicians who manage the postoperative condition of transplant patients be especially sensitive to the possibilities of unexpressed grief. Though these feelings need not be present, a sensitivity to this possibility can be extremely useful in providing a safe and supportive psychological ambience.

The Patient

Once the clinician managing the case of a transplant recipient is sensitized to the possibility that amid all the celebration there is a loss that must be grieved, the task of managing the demands of the new organ can become significantly easier. To begin with, the clinician who understands this process poses a significantly smaller threat to the patient, in comparison to clinicians who have a tendency to judge any emotion other than enthusiasm harshly. Aware that there may be a sense of loss, the clinician provides a milieu of open acceptance that is often crucial to a patient who also has a tendency to judge and/or react to negative emotions with surprise or dismay.

The grief process has a way of evoking a roller coaster-like range of emotions that is extremely threatening to its victims. It is therefore essential that the patient be given every opportunity to express the fullest possible range of emotions and understand that those emotions are well within the boundaries of normalcy when such major bodily restructuring has occurred. Where patients feel uncomfortable with words, nonverbal strategies such as art and music therapy can be highly effective in releasing the flow of confusing emotions, which always seem to be bottled up because of their threatening nature. Where necessary, psychiatric consultation can also be extremely effective. Regardless of the strategy, it is imperative that the patient understand that physiological healing processes are also accompanied by psychological healing processes.

The transition of both mind and body that every transplant procedure represents is by no means the simple and straightforward mechanical process of removing old and worn out parts and replacing them with factory-built replacements. On the contrary, the transition involves a major reorientation from what is often a prolonged presurgical struggle for survival to a postsurgical struggle against biological and psychological "rejection." The body must be aided in providing a suitable host-environment for the new organ, and so must the mind be aided in providing a healthy environment for this biological miracle. In this regard, the grief process forms a rough parallel to the immunological outbursts we know of as tissue rejection. While drugs can work to suppress the immune system's rejection, careful clinical guidance can help the mind's rejection (that we know of as grief) be expressed and reshaped into the positive acceptance of a new existential reality. This is the goal of all grief work.

The Provider

Enlightening the provider with an understanding of the unexpected psychological chaos that can often accompany a transplant recipient is not only a help to the patient, but can also serve to enhance the psychological well-being of the clinician as well. Before information on the nature of the grief process that may accompany organ transplantation was incorporated into the body of literature that now exists, clinicians found themselves disturbed, if not deeply distressed, by the enigmatic self-destructive behavior that cropped up in their patients at a time when celebration and joy were expected. Not only could they not provide an open and trusting environment for their newly troubled patients, the patient's self-destructiveness and neglect were actually causing the physicians to perceive them as enemy.

In this troubled arena, not only the recipients found themselves struggling with strange negative emotions; the physicians sometimes found themselves furious at their patients, yet unable to express their grief (i.e., anger) in any appropriate manner. When grief is either blocked or prevented from being channeled into constructive and nonthreatening expressions, it has a means of spreading its unpleasantness to everyone surrounding those stricken with grief. In these situations, all those who encounter the grief victim find themselves enshrouded in grief. When this "physician grief" can be appropriately channeled, legitimized, and ultimately worked through, it not only helps the physician personally, but also has a profoundly salutary effect on the patient-provider relationship. When it is not appropriately worked through, it can severely disturb the morale of the clinical staff and lead to many stress-ridden consequences, not the least of which can be burnout.

An Integrated Approach to Psychotherapy with the ESRD Population: A Case Presentation

Lissa Parsonnet

Federal funding of the ESRD program, coupled with startling advances in medical technology, have created a population of patients with a complexity of medical and ethical problems not previously encountered. Health care providers are now faced with the need to develop skills rapidly to meet the challenges posed by this new population.

Traditional psychodynamically oriented techniques, emphasizing insight and character change, are often found to be too slow and arduous to meet the needs of the medically ill. Cognitive/behavioral therapy, with its focus on changing cognitions and altering behaviors, makes some clinicians uncomfortable by ignoring intrapsychic processes. This paper will illustrate how an integrative approach to psychotherapy helped an ESRD patient to regain control and autonomy of both his health and his life. This technique is based upon the theory of "therapeutic eclecticism," the process of selecting concepts, methods, and strategies from a variety of current theories that work (Brummer and Shostrum 1982).

CASE PRESENTATION

George was a 58-year-old railroad employee, referred to me by his wife, Sue. George had been widowed after a 35-year marriage. One year later, he married Sue, thus alienating his four grown sons,

Lissa Parsonnet, MS, ACSW, is Oncology/Nephrology Social Worker and Behavioral Consultant, Department of Social Work, Memorial Sloan-Kettering Hospital, New York, NY.

who felt that their mother's memory had been desecrated. Months after his marriage, George was diagnosed with cancer.

Two months into this illness, George was brought to the Intensive Care Unit in acute renal failure, which soon necessitated chronic hemodialysis three times per week. It was at this point that Sue decided that both she and George needed counseling and contacted me. For eight months, George and Sue worked with me as needed, both individually and as a couple. Our work at that time involved an ego supportive approach, aimed at ". . . restoring, maintaining, or enhancing the individual's adapted functioning as well as strengthening or building ego where there are deficits or impairments" (Goldstein 1984).

After eight months, George's condition began to deteriorate rapidly. He became progressively weaker and less able to function. While he continued to receive hemodialysis treatments three times per week, his oncologist felt that there was no longer an appropriate chemotherapy to offer him.

George suddenly presented with a marked change of behavior, displaying an obsessive concern with money. While the couple's financial resources had gradually been depleted throughout the course of his illness, George had left financial matters strictly to Sue, who was an accountant. George now began opening bills, paying some, billing others incorrectly to his insurance company. He reworked the couple's checkbook so that it was incomprehensible either to him or to Sue. He called Sue four to six times a day at work to ask questions about bills, checks, or claims.

When she arrived home from work, George bombarded Sue with a series of questions and concerns about their finances. On two occasions he woke her at night to ask if a certain bill had been reimbursed by their insurance carrier. George discussed nothing else with his wife; this behavior began to carry over to the dialysis unit as well. After four weeks of this, Sue called and came in to discuss this with me. She explained that she was unable to cope with the nonstop financial scrutiny and could not make George understand how his behavior was disturbing her. Sue felt frustrated and strained; she was unable to sleep, eat, or work without interruption from George, always about money. I suggested that we all meet together; we met the following week.

Discussion revealed that George was, in fact, aware that his behavior was pushing his wife away. This upset and hurt him, yet he felt unable to stop. George reported feeling "out-of-control" and unable to gain control of his "financial obsession."

PSYCHODYNAMIC FORMULATION

Freud wrote in *Inhibitions, Symptoms, and Anxiety* that a *symptom* "denotes the presence of some pathological process" (1959, p. 13). He went on to explain that by repression, the ego is able to prevent an idea from becoming conscious. It may find expression through *"displacement,"* a substitution that retains no sense of pleasure and that has "the quality of compulsion" (pp. 17 and 21). Anxiety is experienced in reaction to a perception of danger. *"Symptom formation"* then serves as a means of "avoiding the danger which the anxiety has signalled" (p. 55).

In "The Ego and the Id" (1957), Freud suggested that the fear of death is a development of the fear of castration. Finally, in "Anxiety and Instinctual Life" (1965), Freud symbolically equated *feces* with *money*.

Using classical psychoanalytical theory, we might understand George's symptom, his sudden obsessive concern with money, in the following way: as George's disease progressed, he began to fear that he might not, in fact, survive. Initially this fear occurred on an unconscious level, reawakening castration anxiety and issues of the Oedipal period. This reawakening of Oedipal issues was accompanied by a defense mechanism characteristic of the Oedipal period, in this case, regression. George regressed to the anal stage, characterized by a preoccupation with bowel control, symbolized by money. In other words, George displaced onto money his unconscious fear of death, and the anxiety associated with it. Classical psychoanalytic theory helps us to understand George, but offers only long-term psychoanalysis or psychodynamic psychotherapy with which to treat him. George's prognosis at this time gave him only about six months to live, due to the rapid progression of his cancer. Furthermore, while George was requesting help, he was not requesting a treatment as demanding as psychoanalysis, nor did he have the physical energy to embark upon such a course. This is a common condition when working with the medically ill.

BEHAVIORAL FORMULATION

Behavioral theory would view George's sudden change of behavior very differently. According to such theory, *obsessive thought* is an unwanted thought that intrudes upon a person, bringing fear, depression, or some other disturbance in its wake (Fensterheim and Glazer 1983). *Ruminative obsessions* are thoughts that intrude over and over, bringing anxiety and/or depression in their wake. When a *compulsion* is present, it functions as a negative reinforcer. The compulsion subtracts anxiety and thereby maintains the entire process (Fensterheim and Glazer 1983). In George's case, a ruminative obsession (finances) caused anxiety. His compulsion (constant discussion of money) served to decrease the anxiety and thus maintain the symptom. While this formulation may lead to a more functional treatment plan, it ignores George's progressive illness, and the feelings that such deterioration might evoke. Also omitted is any feeling George might have regarding the estrangement from his sons. This loss was quite painful to George, and represented another area in his life in which he felt out of control.

As the social worker working with this couple, I felt that neither theoretical formulation provided enough insight or guidance to treat this couple's problem. Viewing the situation from *both* perspectives, however, proved quite useful.

INTERVENTION

The initial intervention employed with George was a behavioral technique known as a "Time-Out Technique." In our initial meeting, George, Sue, and I formulated the following assignment for George: he was to discuss his financial concerns with Sue on Fridays from 7:00-9:00 P.M. He was to discuss financial concerns with me on Tuesdays from 10:00-10:30 A.M. Other concerns would be discussed with me Tuesdays from 10:30-11:00 A.M., thus acknowledging that I felt that there were issues beyond finances that would need to be addressed. Financial concerns were not to be discussed with anyone else, or at any other times. Sue agreed to leave the room for 15 minutes should George breach the agreement. The dialysis nurses were apprised of the situation and were very supportive of the effort. In between discussions, George was instructed to write down all of his concerns, so that none would be overlooked.

OUTCOME

George's financial concerns subsided within one week. Relations between George and Sue improved immediately. George then began to address his physical deterioration. He and I formulated questions relevant to his disease, which George posed to his oncologist and nephrologist. He was able to gain an understanding of his medical condition and prognosis. George reported feeling a greater sense of control. The behavioral intervention helped George to face issues, which could then be "worked through" in a psychodynamic sense.

George asked to discontinue dialysis, stating that he did not want to grow progressively weaker and suffer increasing pain, when the certain outcome was death, probably within six months. He considered discontinuing dialysis as a way of controlling his situation, and "meeting his maker in his own way." A psychiatrist was called in and validated his competency to make this decision. Two priests were called who assured him that discontinuing treatment would not constitute suicide in God's eyes.

Finally, George felt able to call his estranged sons; the four met peacefully for the first time since his remarriage. Together they discussed what they would each like to have to remember him by. George called his one remaining friend and said good-bye to him, asking him to be available to Sue. He checked his insurance benefits, making certain that a decision to discontinue dialysis would not compromise the life insurance benefits to which Sue was entitled.

Sue was involved in the decision process and supported George's right to autonomy. She told him that she would miss him deeply, but respected his need to do whatever he thought right. The dialysis nurses were also involved, as George spoke with many of them while reaching his decision. All were supportive of his right to autonomy and assured him that they would take care of him in whatever manner was appropriate to his decision.

George asked to be admitted to the hospital, where he died four days later; Sue was at his side. During his brief hospitalization George was visited by his sons and by each member of the dialysis team. The team was uniformly impressed by the serenity with which George awaited his death.

In the setting of chronic, life-threatening illness, especially those involving the ordinary use of extraordinary measures, new issues are raised for both patients and health care professionals. The integration of varying psychotherapeutic techniques may prove more useful to meet these changes than a rigid adherence to any one theory. Such integration requires the practitioner to be flexible and versatile in both use of skills and use of self. Further exploration of such combinations is warranted.

REFERENCES

Brummer, L. M. and E. L. Shostrom. 1982. *Therapeutic Psychology: Fundamentals of Counseling and Psychotherapy* (4th ed.). Englewood Cliffs, NJ: Prentice-Hall.

Fensterheim, H. and H. Glazer. 1983. *Behavioral Psychotherapy: Basic Principles and Case Studies in an Integrative Clinical Model*. New York: Brunner/Mazel.

Freud, S. 1957. " The Ego and the Id." In J. Rickman, ed. *A General Selection from the Works of Sigmund Freud*. New York: Doubleday and Co., Inc. (Original work published 1923).

Freud, S. 1959. *Inhibitions, Symptoms and Anxiety*. J. Strachey, trans. New York: W. W. Norton and Co., Inc.

Freud, S. 1965. "Anxiety and the Instinctual Life." In *New Introductory Lectures on Psychoanalysis*. J. Strachey, trans. New York: W. W. Norton and Co., Inc.

Goldstein, E. 1984. *Ego Psychology and Social Work Practice*. New York: The Free Press.

Illness Intrusiveness
and the Psychosocial Impact
of End-Stage Renal Disease

Gerald M. Devins

End-stage renal disease (ESRD) and its treatment by dialysis and transplantation are generally believed to introduce significant psychosocial issues and adaptive demands for patients. Among the stressors most commonly identified are the constant threat of death and the potential for reduced life expectancy, dependencies on medical machinery and personnel, and decreased physical strength and stamina. Hemodialysis and continuous ambulatory peritoneal dialysis (CAPD), two of the most common forms of treatment for ESRD (Wyngaarden and Smith 1985), also involve stringent dietary and fluid-intake restrictions, must be accompanied by a complex medical regimen, and require significant time commitments. Many people may be forced to reduce their participation in valued activities and interests (e.g., leisure activities, work, household, and/or school duties). Such intrusions threaten the individual's security and enjoyment of life. They may also contribute to other losses, such as reduced feelings of personal prestige, self-respect, and esteem, and an overall reduction in the perceived quality of life

---

Gerald M. Devins, PhD, is Associate Professor of Psychology and National Health Research Scholar, University of Calgary, Department of Psychiatry, Calgary, Alberta, Canada.

The writing of this chapter was supported in part by the National Health Research and Development Program through a National Health Research Scholar award to Gerald M. Devins. The research reported herein was supported by grants to Dr. Devins from the Alberta Provincial Mental Health Advisory Council and by the National Health Research and Development Program of Health and Welfare Canada.

83

(Binik, Devins, and Orme, in press; Blagg 1978; Czaczkes and De-Nour 1978; Devins in press; Devins et al. 1981, 1983; Johnson, McCauley, and Copley 1982; Kutner, Brogan, and Kutner 1986; Levy 1981a).

Implicit among these stressors is the construct of *illness intrusiveness*, which relates to the extent to which an illness and/or its treatment may interfere with important facets of a person's life. Illness-related disruptions to ongoing interests and activities may occur in ESRD through direct, indirect, or secondary effects. *Direct interference* may be introduced, for example, through the physiological effects of irreversible renal failure, such as reduced physical strength and stamina or increased uremic symptoms (e.g., drowsiness, concentration difficulties, nausea, easy bruising or bleeding) that may limit one's ability to maintain active participation in vocational and avocational domains. Such difficulties are often augmented by the presence of intercurrent nonrenal problems, such as diabetes, bone and cardiovascular disease. Direct interference may also occur when elements of the treatment regimen come into conflict with lifestyles and activity patterns. Dialysis center treatment schedules, for example, may require that a person dialyze during working hours, making it more difficult to maintain full-time employment. *Indirect interference* may be introduced to the extent that family relationships and friendship patterns are disrupted or affected. Following the onset of end-stage kidney failure and the need for treatment by dialysis or transplantation, for example, the perceptions of a person held by family members may change dramatically. The person may come to be fundamentally construed as a "chronically sick" and "helpless" *patient*, whereas he or she may previously have been considered very much an independent and capable individual. Family roles and responsibilities may, thus, begin to shift, with the result that the ESRD patient's autonomy and independence are eroded significantly. Similar effects may also occur within friendships. The nature and frequency of social and leisure activities may thus be disrupted. *Secondary consequences* of decreased involvement in valued activities may introduce additional disruptions or losses. Increased feelings of helplessness and depression among patients, for example, may lead to even further withdrawal from daily patterns of involvements. Sexual dysfunctions may introduce significant challenges to marital adjustment or may simply exacerbate preexisting difficulties.

Understandably, such disruptions are believed to compromise the quality of life in ESRD; this issue has received considerable clinical and research attention (Binik 1983; Binik and Chowanec 1986; Blagg 1978; Cassileth et al. 1984; Devins in press; Evans et al. 1985; Levy 1981b, 1983). This chapter will address the construct of *illness intrusiveness* as it contributes to the psychosocial impact of ESRD upon patients. In attempting to accomplish this, it will be important to distinguish between "objective" and "perceived" intrusiveness, to examine illness-related variables that contribute to these constructs, and to focus on the mechanisms by which these factors impose their effects upon psychosocial well-being and distress.

OBJECTIVE AND PERCEIVED INTRUSIVENESS

As indicated, the situation faced by ESRD patients is characterized by a number of illness-related variables that may introduce barriers or impediments to the continuation of preexisting lifestyles, activities, and interests and thereby contribute to increased illness intrusiveness. It has long been argued, for example, that available renal replacement therapies differ significantly in the intrusions and demands that they impose upon patients, with the result that the psychosocial impact of ESRD is believed to be very much dependent upon the particular form of treatment involved (Evans et al. 1985; Johnson et al. 1982; Rodin et al. 1985; Simmons, Anderson, and Kamstra 1984; Toledo-Pereyra et al. 1985). A naturally occurring continuum of intrusiveness can be identified by ranking the various treatments in terms of (a) the degree to which the schedule of delivery requires that patients relinquish or reschedule valued activities; (b) the amount of time involved; and (c) the stringency of associated dietary and fluid-intake limitations (Devins et al. 1983). In terms of these criteria, hemodialysis seems objectively to be most intrusive: the blood is cleansed extracorporeally by an artificial kidney requiring the patient to remain relatively immobile throughout the process; three weekly four- to eight-hour treatments are usually required; and the associated regimen entails stringent dietary and fluid-intake restrictions plus a variety of medications. Hemodialysis may be performed in a hospital or satellite center (in-center dialysis) or in a patient's own home (home dialysis). In the former, patients may accept primary responsibility for treatment (self-administered), as is the case in home dialysis, or they may relinquish this responsibility to medical personnel (staff-administered incenter dialysis). To the extent that patient involvement in the administration of hemodialysis can decrease the constraints associated with this form of treatment, its degree of intrusiveness may also be reduced (Devins in press). For example, the capability to perform self-administered hemodialysis may mean that treatment sessions can be scheduled so that they conform to a patient's own timetable more closely than can be accomplished when one is dependent upon treatment staff to perform these functions.

CAPD may be less intrusive than hemodialysis: dialysis is performed continuously within one's own body as the patient performs his or her regular schedule of activities. The CAPD regimen typically entails four daily exchanges of dialysate solution, each exchange requiring 30-60 minutes to complete, plus a series of medications and dietary restrictions (generally these restrictions are less limiting than are those associated with hemodialysis). Treatment by CAPD does not require that a patient be immobilized for more than 30-60 minutes at any given time, however, and so it would seem to be less intrusive than treatment by maintenance hemodialysis. Finally, renal transplantation seems least intrusive after the successful completion of surgery, requiring only the daily administration of immunosuppressive, and possibly other, medications, in liquid or tablet form. Once a transplanted kidney has begun to work normally, no particular restrictions are routinely imposed. Thus, in descending order of intrusiveness, an *objective* continuum of illness intrusiveness in ESRD might include: (a) hospital hemodialysis (with staff-administered incenter dialysis possibly more intrusive than self-administered incenter dialysis due to increased patient participation in the latter); (b) home hemodialysis; (c) CAPD; and (d) successful renal transplantation. Similar rankings have been proposed by others (Kutner and Cardenas 1981; Oreopoulos 1980).

It must be acknowledged, however, that this particular continuum is somewhat arbitrary and that several other reasonable alternatives can be constructed. If one were to adopt a criterion of "number of treatments required per week," for example, then CAPD would be considered much more intrusive than hemodialysis, insofar as the former typically involves 28 treatments per week, whereas the latter usually involves only three. A criterion of "degree of family life disruption," on the other hand, might result in home hemodialysis being considered to be most intrusive, followed by CAPD, the two modes of incenter hemodialysis, and lastly, successful renal transplantation. Yet another reasonable criterion might be the "degree to which patients must worry about the continued effectiveness or success of treatment," which would make renal transplantation more intrusive than any form of hemodialysis or CAPD, in that a transplanted kidney can fail at any time and for no apparent reason (Guttmann 1979).

Depending upon the particular criterion adopted, therefore, each of the various forms of treatment for ESRD might be argued to be more or less intrusive than any of the other available treatments. In actuality, it is unlikely that any one of these dimensions, alone, contributes to the intrusiveness of ESRD as it is *perceived* overall by a patient. Moreover, the actual degree of disruption to individual activities and interests may differ substantially, depending on circumstances, values, and lifestyles. Individual differences in personality and coping styles are also likely to influence significantly the degree to which one's health situation impacts upon nonhealth aspects of life (Devins et al. 1986). Our own research (reviewed below) has, indeed, indicated that perceptions of the intrusiveness of ESRD do vary considerably, both among individuals receiving the same form of treatment and across the recipients of different therapeutic modalities. Nevertheless, "objective" and "perceived" intrusiveness have been hypothesized to covary, and each is believed to be importantly related to psychosocial well-being and distress in ESRD (Devins et al. 1983).

DETERMINANTS OF INTRUSIVENESS IN ESRD

Several illness-related variables have been hypothesized to introduce barriers and impediments to ESRD patients' continued involvement in valued activities and interests. Clearly the most commonly identified factor has been the mode of treatment received by an individual. As indicated, hemodialysis has been believed to be most intrusive, renal transplantation least intrusive, with CAPD somewhere between these two extremes. The majority of studies have investigated this issue in the context of a focus on quality of life and the extent to which this may be compromised in ESRD.

Evans et al. (1985), for example, compared "functional impairment," as indicated by the Karnofsky Scale (Karnofsky and Burchenal 1949), and the "ability to work at a job for pay," among other indicators of quality of life, across 859 individuals receiving treatment by incenter ($n = 347$) and home hemodialysis ($n = 287$), CAPD ($n = 81$), as well as posttransplantation ($n = 144$). Participants were sampled from 11 dialysis and transplantation centers throughout the United States and data were obtained via personal interview and chart review procedures. Results indicated that posttransplant patients were characterized by significantly lower levels of impairment and greater ability to work than were patients on any form of dialysis. However, no differences in these variables appeared to emerge among patients receiving any of the three forms of dialysis. Successful renal transplantation, thus, emerged as clearly less intrusive than any of the three forms of dialytic therapy but no further differences in intrusiveness appeared to be indicated.

Simmons et al. (1984) compared measures of physical and emotional well-being among 70 people receiving treatment by incenter hemodialysis, 251 on CAPD, and 82 with a successfully functioning kidney transplant. Participants on hemodialysis had been selected from seven different centers throughout midwestern America. CAPD participants were sampled randomly from a larger pool of individuals ($N = 504$) who had been recruited for a national study (involving a total of 187 different treatment centers across the United States), although no explanation was provided as to why a CAPD patient subset of this particular size should be extracted for these analyses. The posttransplant patients had been selected from a single midwestern facility. Data were obtained via a mail-back questionnaire methodology. Of particular relevance to the issue of treatment modality differences in the intrusiveness of ESRD, Simmons et al. compared these three treatment groups in terms of the "lack of difficulty in daily activities" as indicated by self-report, the proportions of participants who were currently working or in school, and the numbers of days in hospital. Successful transplant recipients reported that they experienced significantly less difficulty with daily activities than did either hemodialysis or CAPD patients. However, no difference was noted between the two dialysis groups. Similarly, a significantly higher proportion of posttransplant patients were working or in school as compared to the two dialysis groups. A higher proportion of CAPD as compared to hemodialysis patients were also employed or enrolled in school; however, this difference did not reach conventional levels of statistical significance. Finally, none of the three treatments appeared to be significantly different in terms of the numbers of days for which patients had been hospitalized.

Johnson et al. (1982) also compared several quality of life indicators relating to the intrusiveness of ESRD among four different groups, including patients (a) on hemodialysis with no previous history of transplantation awaiting cadaveric transplantation ($n = 10$), (b) on maintenance hemodialysis with no previous history of transplantation and not awaiting a transplant ($n = 19$), (c) transplanted successfully with cadaveric grafts ($n = 20$), and (d) with failed cadaveric transplants who had returned to hemodialysis ($n = 10$). A total of 19 "objective" and "subjective" indicators of life quality were obtained and compared across these groups. Measures relevant to illness intrusiveness included: perceived (a) "ease" and (b) "freedom" in one's present life; (c) number of activities or sports given up because of ESRD; (d) employment status; (e) number of days in hospital during the preceding 12 months; (f) number of hours required for treatment during the preceding week; and (g) feelings of fatigue. A mail-back questionnaire procedure was employed. Clearly, the most consistent pattern of differences involved the comparison of patients with a failed transplant as compared to those whose new kidneys had continued to function. As compared to failed transplant recipients who had been forced to return to maintenance hemodialysis, individuals with a successful transplant reported significantly higher levels of ease and freedom in their lives, required less hours per week for treatment, and were hospitalized for fewer days in the preceding year. They were also significantly more likely to be employed on a full-time basis (including "housework") and reported significantly lower levels of fatigue. These two groups did not differ, however, in the numbers of activities or sports that they had given up due to ESRD or in part-time employment status. There were only two corresponding differences between dialysis patients who had not experienced the failure of a transplanted kidney and successful transplant recipients: (a) greater feelings of freedom in one's present life and (b) lower levels of fatigue were reported by posttransplant patients. No other significant differences were observed. Finally, no differences emerged between the failed transplant and dialysis (i.e., no transplant attempt) patient groups for any of these measures. Thus, very few differences were observed between the dialysis (no transplant failure) and transplant groups and none occurred between the two dialysis groups. The major difference appears to have occurred between the failed and successful transplant groups. Insofar as the former patients were also in significantly poorer health than were any of the others, it would appear that generally poor nonrenal health may be an important contributor to the intrusiveness of ESRD (cf. Binik and Devins 1986).

The *perceived intrusiveness* of ESRD has also been examined directly in two studies conducted by my colleagues and myself. In the first study (Devins et al. 1983), a sample of 70 ESRD patients on incenter staff-administered ($n = 14$), incenter self-administered ($n = 12$), and home hemodialysis ($n = 9$), CAPD ($n = 10$), and posttransplantation ($n = 25$) participated in a standardized interview in which measures of the perceived intrusiveness of ESRD, depression, normal positive and negative moods, self-esteem, and somatic symptoms of distress were obtained. Of particular relevance to the issue of the intrusiveness of ESRD and the continuum of treatments hypothesized above, was the instrument that was developed to assess perceived intrusiveness. Participants were asked to provide ratings of the degree to which "ESRD and/or its treatment interferes with" 11 aspects of life that had been identified in previous research as importantly related to the perceived quality of life (Flanagan 1978). Ratings were made along a 7-point scale, ranging from "not very much" to "very much" and the following aspects of life were included: work, financial security and material need satisfaction, recreation, family and marital relations, other social relations, sex, self-expression, religious expression, community and civic activities, health, and diet. These ratings were then summed to provide an overall perceived intrusiveness score and were compared across the five patient groups. Corresponding ratings were obtained for each participant from hospital staff and significant others (e.g., spouse). The results indicated that patients' perceived intrusiveness did, indeed, differ significantly as a function of treatment modality. Consistent with the continuum of treatment modalities proposed above, posttransplant patients perceived this form of treatment to be significantly less intrusive than did patients on all forms of dialysis, combined—i.e., CAPD and the three modes of hemodialysis. However, no significant difference was observed in perceived intrusiveness across individuals receiving any of the forms of hemodialysis or CAPD. These results were corroborated by the corresponding ratings that had been obtained from hospital staff members and from significant others.

This pattern of findings was replicated in a second study (Devins et al. 1987). A new sample of 100 ESRD patients on incenter ($n = 36$) and home ($n = 16$) hemodialysis, CAPD ($n = 11$), and posttransplantation ($n = 37$) was selected. A standardized interview was administered and included a battery of measures similar to that employed in the preceding study. Once again, perceived intrusiveness was compared across the four treatment groups and a similar pattern of differences was observed. Posttransplant patients evidenced significantly lower levels of perceived intrusiveness as compared to individuals on dialysis. Again, however, no difference was observed in the perceived intrusiveness of ESRD and/or its treatment among individuals receiving treatment by incenter or home hemodialysis or via CAPD. Thus, although the various forms of treatment currently employed in ESRD do differ in the extent to which they introduce disruptions to ongoing activities and interests, they do not appear to do so in as consistent a fashion as has generally been believed.

In anticipation of this, our second study also included a number of more specific variables that were hypothesized to contribute to the perceived intrusiveness of ESRD. These included: (a) elevated levels of uremic symptoms (e.g., muscle cramps, easy bruising and bleeding, "restless legs"); (b) the presence of intercurrent nonrenal health problems (e.g., cardiac, respiratory, or bone disease); (c) difficulties in performing daily activities, such as walking and climbing stairs; (d) the amounts of time taken up by ESRD and its treatment; and (e) specific illness-related concerns (e.g., that one might die because of ESRD). Each of these factors was hypothesized to contribute to increased perceived intrusiveness. Moreover, in an attempt to provide an initial test of the causal priorities among these variables, data were collected on two different occasions, separated by a constant lag of six weeks. Multiple regression (path) analyses, controlling for initial levels of perceived intrusiveness, indicated that initial levels of four of these variables significantly predicted subsequent increases in perceived intrusiveness six weeks later. Elevated initial levels of uremic symptoms, difficulties in performing daily activities, time taken up by treatment, and illness-related concerns, each contributed uniquely and independently to subsequent significant increases in the perceived intrusiveness of ESRD. However, initial levels of perceived intrusiveness also significantly predicted subsequent levels of two of these hypothesized determinants—difficulties in daily activities and illness-related concerns—suggesting that these particular relationships may be either nonrecursive in nature or simply spurious, attributable to a "third" variable (Cook and Campbell 1979; Kenny 1979). When compared across patients receiving incenter and home hemodialysis, CAPD, and renal transplantation, significant differences were observed for each of the five hypothesized determinants. In each case, however, only one pairwise comparison emerged as clearly significant—incenter hemodialysis versus successful renal transplantation.

A reanalysis of some of the data collected in the Devins et al. (1983) study has indicated that perceived intrusiveness levels do not differ significantly (a) between hemodialysis patients who have experienced the failure of a transplanted kidney and those who have not or (b) between successful transplant recipients and dialysis patients, regardless of whether or not they have previously experienced the failure of a transplanted kidney (Binik and Devins 1986).

Finally, although not addressed to the issue of differential intrusions across therapeutic modalities, Sherwood (1983) has reported an investigation of the "impact of renal failure" and its treatment on 11 areas of life among a random sample of 55 incenter hemodialysis patients. The life domains examined included eating habits, leisure time pursuits, sexual activity, social contacts, family relationships, vacation activities, friendships, employment activities, self-esteem, sense of security, and the ability to enjoy life. An interview procedure was employed. Results indicated that a majority of respondents ($\geq$ 53 percent of the entire sample) identified five areas of life as "greatly or moderately affected as a result of becoming a dialysis patient" (p. 56). In descending frequency of identification, these areas included: (a) employment activities; (b) vacation activities; (c) leisure time pursuits; (d) eating habits; and (e) sexual activity. Sherwood also investigated the extent to which the overall "impact" of ESRD on all 11 areas of life, combined, might be related to nonadherence to the hemodialysis regimen. However, no significant relationship was observed.

In summary, these findings collectively support the assertion that the construct of illness intrusiveness is an important component of the psychosocial impact of ESRD. That this construct entails separate objective and perceived dimensions is supported by the fact that patient perceptions of the intrusiveness of ESRD and its treatment do not map neatly and isomorphically onto any a priori continuum that might be constructed on the basis of objective differences among treatment modalities. Although a number of objective facets may differ across the treatments currently available for ESRD, the findings reviewed above have indicated that the various forms of hemodialysis and CAPD do not differ appreciably in the extent to which they may effectively introduce disruptions to patients' lifestyles, valued activities, and interests. Dialysis of any kind, however, appears to be more intrusive than is successful renal transplantation. In addition to treatment modality differences, a number of other illness-related factors have been identified that contribute to the perceived intrusiveness of ESRD. These include: (a) elevated levels of uremic symptoms; (b) intercurrent nonrenal illnesses; (c) difficulties in performing daily activities; (d) increased time requirements; and (e) illness-related concerns.

INTRUSIVENESS AND PSYCHOSOCIAL WELL-BEING AND DISTRESS IN ESRD

While the issue of whether the various renal replacement therapies impose differential psychosocial burdens upon recipients has been the subject of considerable debate, empirical research efforts have been directed at comparing the "quality of life" associated with each (cf. Binik 1983; Binik and Chowanec 1986, for excellent reviews). Quality of life comparisons across the various modes of treatment cannot provide valid results relevant to this issue, however. This is because a number of demographic (e.g., age), psychological (e.g., intelligence), social (e.g., social supports), and medical characteristics (e.g., intercurrent nonrenal conditions) are typically taken into consideration in the assignment of patients to specific forms of treatment. As a result, one cannot rule out the competing hypothesis that quality of life differences across treatment modalities may be attributable to any or all of these confounded differences rather than due to differences in the intrusiveness of the particular modalities in question (Binik 1983; Devins et al. 1983, 1986; Evans et al. 1985; Smith, Hong, Province, and Robson 1985). Moreover, given widespread individual differences in terms of personal resources and coping capabilities, it is not at all clear that differences in quality of life or in psychosocial adjustment can be attributed exclusively to differences in the objective intrusions imposed by a given form of treatment. Few studies have included controls for such differences while simultaneously providing a direct examination of the degree to which differences in psychosocial well-being or distress may be attributable to differences in the intrusiveness associated with each mode of treatment.

In one of the few studies to control for such "case mix" characteristics, Evans et al. (1985) examined the degree of correspondence between subjective and objective quality of life indicators and observed a moderate correlation ($r = .42$, $p < .05$) between functional impairment and a composite variable, including psychological affect, emotional well-being, and life satisfaction. This would appear to support the assertion that objective and perceived intrusiveness covary, but that they are, nevertheless, conceptually distinct. To the best of my knowledge, the relationship between the perceived intrusiveness of ESRD and its psychosocial impact has been examined only in the two studies, noted above, by my colleagues and myself (Devins et al. 1983, 1987).

In the first of these (Devins et al. 1983), nine separate measures of positive and negative moods, life happiness, self-esteem, depression, and somatic symptoms of distress were obtained and were reduced via principal-components factor analysis to two factor scores, corresponding to negative and positive moods, that served as criterion variables. Analyses of partial variance, controlling for age, general nonrenal health, and defensive response styles, indicated that the perceived intrusiveness of ESRD and its treatment was significantly related to both positive and negative moods. Increased levels of perceived intrusiveness were associated with decreased positive and increased negative moods. The same analytic scheme was employed to compare mood levels across patients receiving treatment by staff-administered incenter, self-administered incenter, and home hemodialysis, CAPD, as well as successful transplant recipients. Significant group differences were observed for positive but not for negative moods. Posthoc analyses indicated that posttransplant patients had reported significantly higher levels of positive moods than had patients receiving any form of hemodialysis or CAPD. There were no differences in the levels of positive mood across the four forms of dialysis, however. Thus, the perceived intrusiveness of ESRD and its treatment did appear to relate importantly to psychosocial well-being and distress among patients. Differences in psychosocial well-being and distress across treatment modalities did not display the same pattern, although the finding of differences in positive moods between posttransplant and dialysis patients, combined, did conform to our findings regarding treatment group differences in perceived intrusiveness.

These findings were replicated and extended in our second study (Devins et al. 1987). A broader battery of 14 psychosocial indicators was administered, including the same nine scales that had been employed in the preceding study plus additional measures of hope, nonpathological negative moods, and somatic symptoms of distress. As in the preceding study, these 14 measures were reduced via principal-components analysis to a smaller number of factor scores that could be used as criterion variables. Because of the expanded battery, a three-factor solution was obtained (as compared to the two-factor one extracted in our previous study). Consistent with our previous results, two of these factors corresponded quite closely to nonpathological positive and negative affect. The third factor involved a combination of somatic symptoms and psychiatric depression scales. This factor thus appeared to correspond relatively closely to somatic symptoms of distress, possibly representing those symptoms that have been identified as overlapping between depression and uremia (Devins et al. 1986; Kutner, Fair, and Kutner 1985; Schreiner 1959). The perceived intrusiveness of ESRD was measured via an expanded version of the self-report instrument that had been used in our previous study.

Because data were collected from the same sample of participants on two occasions, separated by a constant lag of six weeks, it was possible to explore in a preliminary way whether the relationship that we had observed between perceived intrusiveness and psychosocial well-being and distress in our initial study was causal or spurious in nature. This was accomplished via a path analysis in which we examined the predictive relationships between the two sets of variables (i.e., perceived intrusiveness and psychosocial well-being and distress). Residualized post-scores (Cohen and Cohen 1983) were employed as the criterion variables in each case so that we could examine the extent to which initial levels of a predictor variable were predictive of *changes* in the criterion of interest (e.g., the extent to which initial levels of perceived intrusiveness were predictive of subsequent changes in psychosocial well-being and distress six weeks later). Statistical controls were also introduced for confounded background and medical variables that were significantly correlated with the psychosocial measures: age, hours worked per week, recent negative and positive life events, and social networks. The issue of whether the relationship is causal or spurious was examined by testing both the hypothesized (e.g., perceived intrusiveness predicts changes in psychosocial well-being) and counter-hypothesized (e.g., psychosocial well-being predicts changes in perceived intrusiveness) path models (Kenny 1979).

As observed in our previous study, the results indicated that the perceived intrusiveness of ESRD was significantly related to psychosocial impact. Consistent with our original finding, relatively high initial levels of perceived intrusiveness significantly predicted reduced levels of positive affect six weeks later, suggesting that perceived intrusiveness may be one important causal factor in the determination of psychosocial well-being in ESRD. Our initial results had also indicated that increased levels of perceived intrusiveness were associated with increased levels of depression and negative affect. This finding was only partially replicated, however. In testing the hypothesized path model, initial levels of perceived intrusiveness were statistically unrelated to (a) somatic and depressive symptoms and (b) relatively normal negative moods. In testing the counter-hypothesized model, however, it became evident that relatively elevated initial levels of somatic-depressive symptoms were actually predictive of subsequent increases in patient perceptions of the intrusiveness of ESRD. Patient perceptions of the intrusiveness of ESRD may, thus, actually be the *product* of somatic-depressive symptoms. Perceived intrusiveness was simply unrelated to nonpathological negative affect, failing to support the hypothesis that these two variables are related at all. Thus, whereas perceived intrusiveness may contribute causally to positive affect and psychosocial well-being among ESRD patients, it would appear actually to represent an *effect* of elevated somatic symptoms and may not be related to negative affect.

Finally, comparisons of positive and negative affect and of somatic-depressive symptoms across recipients on the four treatment modalities indicated a pattern of results that was similar to that observed in our preceding study. Once again only a single statistically significant difference emerged: successful posttransplant patients were characterized by significantly higher levels of positive affect than were patients on incenter or home hemodialysis or CAPD. No reliable difference in positive mood was apparent across hemodialysis or CAPD patients and there were no differences whatsoever across any of the treatment groups in terms of negative affect or somatic-depressive symptoms. These findings further corroborate the suggestion, above, that the fundamental difference in intrusiveness across currently available renal replacement therapies is between successful renal transplantation and all forms of dialysis, combined.

While these results are obviously in need of replication and extension, it is reasonable to speculate that the significance of illness intrusiveness may be more in terms of its impact upon psychosocial well-being and positive affect than in terms of its contributions to depression or distress. It is well established, for example, that positive and negative affect correspond more closely to two independent unipolar dimensions of emotion as opposed to a single bipolar one (Bradburn 1969; Diener 1984). Thus, the impact of increased illness intrusiveness—i.e., a reduction in participation in valued activities and increased impediments to the pursuit of important interests—may contribute to decreases in positive affect and life satisfaction without necessarily influencing negative affect states directly (Costa and McCrae 1980). Depression and psychosocial distress among ESRD patients may derive from problems in living that are quite independent of the illness and/or its treatment (e.g., family and marital, vocational, or economic difficulties, independent stressful life events, or chronic difficulties).

On the other hand, there is a large body of evidence to suggest the contrary—i.e., that a reduction in positively valued experiences and outcomes does contribute importantly to the onset and maintenance of depression and psychosocial distress (Devins et al. 1982; Garber and Seligman 1980; Lewinsohn, Youngren, and Grosscup 1979). While it is possible that depression and negative affect are the products of a qualitatively separate psychosocial mechanism in the ESRD situation, it is also conceivable that depressive symptoms do not begin to emerge until after the illness situation has become extremely restrictive—e.g., to the point where the occurrence of positive experiences has been almost completely eliminated. To the extent that the particular sample of patients that participated in this second study may not have included a sufficient number of individuals whose illness situation had become so restrictive that they were unable to obtain a minimum or "threshold" frequency or quality of positive experiences, it is possible that the experiment may not have achieved sufficient statistical power to detect a relationship between perceived intrusiveness and negative affect. Research currently in progress is continuing to investigate these questions.

CONCLUSIONS AND IMPLICATIONS

ESRD and its treatment can be highly stressful via direct, indirect, and secondary effects upon a patient's lifestyle and the ability to pursue important life goals. The construct of illness intrusiveness relates to illness-related barriers and disruptions to valued activities and interests and has been hypothesized to contribute to decreased psychosocial well-being and increased distress in ESRD. The research reviewed above has indicated that separate objective and perceived dimensions of illness intrusiveness appear to comprise distinct facets of this construct and that each is importantly related to the psychosocial impact experienced by individual patients. In terms of an objective dimension of intrusiveness, the fundamental difference would appear to be between successful renal transplantation and dialytic therapy of any form—incenter staff-administered hemodialysis, incenter self-administered hemodialysis, home hemodialysis or CAPD—with transplantation being consistently less intrusive than dialysis. Findings to date have also indicated that perceived intrusiveness may be an important causal element in the determination of psychosocial well-being or positive affect in ESRD. Results have been less consistent regarding the relation between intrusiveness and psychosocial distress. It will be important for future research to investigate more fully the nature and mechanisms by which illness intrusiveness contributes to the psychosocial impact of ESRD.

Despite the tentativeness with which these results must be viewed, it may be possible clinically to minimize psychosocial difficulties by attempting to reduce illness intrusiveness as it affects the patient. One means of doing this may be to acknowledge during patient education efforts that treatment modality differences do not appear to be as important to psychosocial adaptation as has been emphasized in the past. Health care professionals must do their best to avoid the communication of biases regarding psychosocial advantages and disadvantages of one form of treatment over others, insofar as differences in psychosocial responses may simply be attributable to individual differences among patients in nonrenal or nontreatment factors (e.g., personal resources and strengths, social and financial resources, general nonrenal health). The elimination of such messages may help to prevent the occurrence of "self-fulfilling prophecies" that life on dialysis will be associated with increased feelings of helplessness and depression, for example. It is also important to encourage patients to remain as actively involved as possible in valued activities and to support them in attempting to maintain their involvements in outside interests. Such encouragement and support can help to prevent the occurrence of unnecessary disruptions. Patients, their spouses, and other family members should also be educated about the importance of minimizing disruptions to activity patterns. Thus, communication, education, and "psychosocial management" can help to minimize the extent to which ESRD introduces stressful intrusions into a patient's life and can, thus, also help to facilitate an effective response to the psychosocial issues and adaptive demands imposed by this chronic life-threatening condition.

REFERENCES

Binik, Y.M. 1983. "Coping with Life-threatening Illness: Psychosocial Perspectives on End-stage Renal Disease." *Canadian Journal of Behavioural Science* 15:373-391.

Binik, Y.M. and G.D. Chowanec. 1986. "Quality of Life." In M. Garovoy and R.D. Guttmann, eds. *Renal Transplantation*. New York: Churchill Livingstone, pp. 341-353.

Binik, Y.M. and G.M. Devins. 1986. "Transplant Failure Does Not Compromise Quality of Life in End-stage Renal Disease." *International Journal of Psychiatry in Medicine* 16:281-292.

Binik, Y.M., G.M. Devins, and C.M. Orme. (in press). "Psychological Stress and Coping in End-stage Renal Disease." In R.W.J. Neufeld, ed. *Advances in Investigation of Psychological Stress*. New York: Wiley.

Blagg, C.R. 1978. "Objective Quantification of Rehabilitation in Dialysis and Transplantation." In E.A. Friedman, ed. *Strategy in Renal Failure*. New York: Wiley Interscience, pp. 415-433.

Bradburn, N.M. 1969. *The Structure of Psychological Well-being*. Chicago: Aldine.

Cassileth, B.R., E.J. Lusk, T.B. Strouse, D.S. Miller, L.L. Brown, P.A. Cross and A.N. Tenaglia. 1984. "Psychosocial Status in Chronic Illness: A Comparative Analysis of Six Diagnostic Groups." *New England Journal of Medicine* 311:506-511.

Cohen, J. and P. Cohen. 1983. *Applied Multiple Regression/Correlation Analysis for the Behavioral Sciences* (2nd ed.). Hillsdale, NJ: Erlbaum.

Cook, T.D. and D.T. Campbell. 1979. *Quasi-experimentation: Design and Analysis Issues for Field Settings*. Boston: Houghton Mifflin.

Costa, P.T. and R.R. McCrae. 1980. "Influence of Extraversion and Neuroticism on Subjective Well-being: Happy and Unhappy People. *Journal of Personality and Social Psychology* 38:668-678.

Czaczkes, J.W. and A.K. De-Nour. 1978. *Chronic Hemodialysis as a Way of Life*. New York: Brunner/Mazel.

Devins, G.M. (in press). "Enhancing Personal Control and Minimizing Illness

Intrusiveness." In N.G. Kutner, D.D. Cardenas, and J.D. Bower, eds. *Maximizing Rehabilitation in Chronic Renal Disease*. New York: Pergamon.

Devins, G.M., Y.M. Binik, P. Gorman, M. Dattel, B. McCloskey, G. Oscar, and J. Briggs. 1982. "Perceived Self-efficacy, Outcome Expectations, and Negative Mood States in End-stage Renal Disease." *Journal of Abnormal Psychology* 91:241-244.

Devins, G.M., Y.M. Binik, D.J. Hollomby, P.E. Barre, and R.D. Guttmann. 1981. "Helplessness and Depression in End-stage Renal Disease." *Journal of Abnormal Psychology* 90:531-545.

Devins, G.M., Y.M. Binik, T.A. Hutchinson, D.J. Hollomby, P.E. Barre, and R.D. Guttmann. 1983. "The Emotional Impact of End-stage Renal Disease." *International Journal of Psychiatry in Medicine* 3:327-343.

Devins, G.M., Y.M. Binik, H. Mandin, E.D. Burgess, K. Taub, P.K. Letourneau, S. Buckle, and G.L. Low. 1986. "Denial as a Defense Against Depression in End-stage Renal Disease." *International Journal of Psychiatry in Medicine* 16:151-162.

Devins, G.M., H. Mandin, R.B. Hons, E.D. Burgess, J. Klassen, K. Taub, S. Schorr, P.K. Letourneau, and S. Buckle. 1987. *Determinants and Psychosocial Impact of Illness Intrusiveness in End-stage Renal Disease*. Manuscript submitted for publication.

Diener, E. 1984. Subjective Well-being. *Psychological Bulletin* 95:542-575.

Evans, R.G., D.L. Manninen, L.P. Garrison, L.G. Hart, C.R. Blagg, R.A. Gutman, A.R. Hull, and E.G. Lowrie. 1985. "The Quality of Life of Patients with End-stage Renal Disease." *New England Journal of Medicine* 312:553-559.

Flanagan, J.C. 1978. "Measurement of Quality of Life: Current State of the Art." *Archives of Physical and Rehabilitation Medicine* 63:56-59.

Garber, J. and M.E.P. Seligman, eds. 1980. *Human Helplessness; Theory and Applications*. New York: Academic Press.

Guttmann, R.D. 1979. "Renal Transplantation." *New England Journal of Medicine* 301:975-982; 1038-1048.

Johnson, J.P., C.R. McCauley, and J.B. Copley. 1982. "The Quality of Life of Hemodialysis and Transplant Patients. *Kidney International* 22:286-291.

Karnofsky, D.A. and J.H. Burchenal. 1949. "The Clinical Evaluation of Chemotherapeutic Agents in Cancer." In C.M. MacLeod, ed. *Evaluation of Chemotherapeutic Agents* New York, Columbia Press.

Kenny, D.A. 1979. *Correlation and Causality*. New York: Wiley.

Kutner, N.G., D. Brogan, and M.H. Kutner. 1986. "End-stage Renal Disease Treatment Modality and Patients' Quality of Life." *American Journal of Nephrology* 6:396-402.

Kutner, N.G. and D.D. Cardenas. 1981. "Rehabilitation Status of Chronic Renal Disease Patients Undergoing Dialysis: Variations by Age Category." *Archives of Physical and Rehabilitation Medicine* 62:626-630.

Kutner, N.G., P.L. Fair, and M.H. Kutner. 1985. "Assessing Depression and Anxiety in Chronic Dialysis Patients." *Journal of Psychosomatic Research* 29:23-31.

Levy, N.B. 1981a. "Psychological Reactions to Machine Dependency: Hemodialysis." *Psychiatric Clinics of North America* 4:351-363.

Levy, N.B., ed. 1981b. *Psychonephrology 1: Psychological Factors in Hemodialysis and Transplantation*. New York: Plenum.

Levy, N.B. ed. 1983. *Psychonephrology 2: Psychological Problems in Kidney Failure and Their Treatment*. New York: Plenum.

Lewinsohn, P.M., M.A. Youngren, and S.J. Grosscup. 1979. "Reinforcement and Depression." In R.A. Depue, ed. *The Psychobiology of the Depressive Disorders*. New York: Academic Press.

Oreopoulos, D.G. 1980. "An Update on the Continuous Ambulatory Peritoneal Dialysis (CAPD)." *International Journal of Artificial Organs* 3:231-234.

Rodin, G., K. Voshart, D. Cattran, P. Halloran, C. Cardella, and S. Fenton. 1985. "Cadaveric Renal Transplant Failure: The Short-term Sequelae." *International Journal of Psychiatry in Medicine* 15:357-364.

Schreiner, G.C. 1959. "Mental and Personality Changes in the Uremic Syndrome." *Medical Annals of the District of Columbia* 28:316-324.

Sherwood, R.J. 1983. "The Impact of Renal Failure and Dialysis Treatments on Patients' Lives and on Their Compliance Behavior." In N.B. Levy, ed. *Psychonephrology 2: Psychological Problems in Kidney Failure and Their Treatment*. New York: Plenum.

Simmons, R.G., C. Anderson, and L. Kamstra. 1984. "Comparison of Quality of Life of Patients on Continuous Ambulatory Peritoneal Dialysis, Hemodialysis, and After Transplantation." *American Journal of Kidney Diseases* 4:253-255.

Smith, M.C., B.A. Hong, M.A. Province, and A.M. Robson. 1985. "Does Social Support Determine the Treatment Setting for Hemodialysis Patients?" *American Journal of Kidney Diseases* 5:27-31.

Toledo-Pereyra, L.H., A. Schneider, S. Baskin, L. McNichol, K. Thavarajah, W.J. Lin, and J. Whitten. 1985. "Rehabilitation After Dialysis and Kidney Transplantation." *Boletin d'Asociacion Medica de Puerto-Rico* 77:227-230.

Wyngaarden, J.B. and L.H. Smith, eds. 1985. *Cecil Textbook of Medicine* (17th ed.). Philadelphia, W.B. Saunders.

Helping Patients Cope with the Loss of a Renal Transplant

Ramaswamy Viswanathan

Renal transplantation is truly a gift of life. Apart from providing a patient who has end-stage renal disease (ESRD) with a way to continue living, it promotes more independent functioning than with hemodialysis, and increases the free time available to the individual (Abram and Buchanan 1976-77; Levy 1986). Hence, renal transplantation is becoming an increasingly popular option, and is becoming more widely available. At the State University of New York Health Science Center at Brooklyn (SUNY HSCB), formerly known as Downstate Medical Center, about 150 renal transplantations are performed per year, one-third of which are from living related donors. Even though the recent advent of cyclosporine has significantly improved the transplant survival rates, rejection is still a reality. At SUNY HSCB, the one-year survival rate of a renal homograft is about 75-80 percent for cadaveric transplants, and about 90 percent for living related donor transplants (LRDT). Thus, while the high success rate is encouraging, there is a significant number of people who have to cope with the trauma of the loss of the transplanted kidney. This paper deals with the stressors faced by such individuals and how they can be helped to cope with them.

STRESSORS ASSOCIATED WITH THE LOSS OF A RENAL TRANSPLANT

Rejection or the threat of rejection of a transplanted kidney results in a period of emotional turmoil for the individual, as he or

Ramaswamy Viswanathan, MD, DMSc, is Clinical Associate Professor of Psychiatry, and is Associate Director, Psychiatric Consultation-Liaison Service, State University of New York Health Science Center, Brooklyn, NY.

she is reacting to a number of losses and other stressors as outlined below:

Loss of a cherished form of treatment. For many people a major reason for choosing renal transplantation is their view that transplantation is a more desirable form of treatment compared to dialysis (Abram and Buchanan 1976-77; Freyberger 1983; Nadel and Clark 1986). Hence, when the transplantation fails, there is despondency that a highly valued treatment has failed. While patients can continue to live, thanks to dialysis, and in fact many patients feel thankful for this (Streltzer et al. 1983-84), some find it difficult to adapt to hemodialysis, as they perceive it as a more demanding form of treatment and are unable to accept the limitations in life imposed by it (Abram and Buchanan 1976-77; Johnson et al. 1982). Dependence on others for hemodialysis, restrictions on one's schedule and work opportunities, some physical effects of hemodialysis, and the fact of being dependent on a machine are not tolerated well by some people (Gulledge et al. 1983). Our clinical experience suggests that people who did not have much exposure to hemodialysis prior to their transplantation find it especially hard to adapt to hemodialysis later.

Losing an object of attachment. In transplantation, there is a psychological process of incorporation and assimilation of the transplanted foreign organ into one's own body image, making it one's own (Castelnuovo-Tedesco 1978). During this process one forms an attachment to the organ. Generally, the longer one has had the successful transplant, the greater the attachment. Personality variables play an important role in the intensity of the attachment. The more intense the attachment, the deeper is the sorrow at the loss.

Guilt at having wasted the donated kidney. This is especially strong with LRDT. The guilt is even more acute if the transplantation had deprived another family member also suffering from renal failure of a potential LRDT, as in the case of some familial renal diseases.

Guilt or shame at failing the expectations of others. The patient may perceive the disappointments of family, friends, and staff, and may react with a sense of personal responsibility and failure.

Uncertainty, prolonged hospitalization, and physical complications. In the case of chronic rejection, the prolonged uncertainty about whether the kidney can be saved can itself be emotionally taxing, as is the prolonged hospitalization. Physical complications due to the rejection process, due to the aggressive immunosuppressive treatment to reverse the rejection process, or due to intercurrent illness (e.g., fatigue, infections, steroid-induced affective disorder, complications of diabetes mellitus) can put considerable stress on the patient.

Loss of sense of control. One has a need to feel in control of one's body and environment (Beiber 1980). When this is threatened or lost, severe emotional distress, a sense of helplessness, anxiety, and depression may ensue (Viswanathan and Kachur 1986; Viswanathan and Vizner 1984).

HELPING PATIENTS COPE

An understanding of the nature of coping mechanisms can help one devise ways of helping a patient to cope with the trauma of renal transplant rejection. Many of the principles are similar to coping with other acute and chronic illnesses with significant losses (Viswanathan 1988). Coping can be broadly divided into instrumental and palliative mechanisms (Monat and Lazarus 1977). Instrumental coping involves taking action to change the situation. Palliative coping involves changing one's perception of the situation. (It is analogous to obtaining pain relief by taking an analgesic medication.) Both kinds of coping are required in most cases. It is important to help patients develop a "coping orientation" instead of just feeling helpless.

Instrumental Coping

Whenever possible, instrumental coping should be encouraged. Being compliant with treatment recommendations and pursuing another renal transplantation are two examples of instrumental coping. Patients who view hemodialysis as too restrictive should be made aware of the very productive lives led by many hemodialysis patients, and should be encouraged to actively explore means of pursuing their goals despite being on hemodialysis. Continuous ambulatory peritoneal dialysis (CAPD) is another means for patients to have more freedom of movement and independence. Home dialysis may give patients greater flexibility and sense of control (Rabin 1983).

Palliative Coping

When the rejection can not be reversed, one has to be enabled to accept the loss. Even when rejection is partial and there is the possibility that it can be reversed, palliative coping is still needed to reduce emotional distress during the recovery process. In many instances palliative coping reduces emotional distress and helps the individual concentrate his or her energies on instrumental coping. In some instances, some kinds of palliative coping can be maladaptive by interfering with instrumental coping (for example, a patient ignores hematuria or flank pain, uses denial ("everything is fine") and does not seek medical help). The following are some examples of palliative coping that are useful in helping patients cope with renal transplant rejection:

Buying time. In my inpatient consultation work, I find this a very valuable approach when I am called to see patients with acute loss who are very demoralized. Such patients have to be helped to maintain hope and patience. When patients refuse hemodialysis and other treatment following a renal transplant rejection, asking them to try out the treatment for a specified period of time and see how things work out, and pointing out that they always have the option to withdraw from treatment later, often remarkably improve the patients' mood and willingness to engage in treatment. Basically one is asking patients to subject themselves to life experiences for a period of time to develop a more realistic perspective on their problems. It also gives time for healing and coping mechanisms to evolve, and gives time for psychotherapeutic interventions.

Hope. Hope is important for a person to engage in coping and treatment, and to reduce emotional distress. One has to encourage hope, taking care to see that the expectations are realistic, in order to avoid the negative effects of later disappointments. Seeing or learning about others who have coped successfully with similar problems can be enormously helpful. Hope is important when helping patients cope with a protracted period of uncertainty, as when they have a partial rejection and it is not clear whether their transplant can ultimately be saved or not. Religious patients should be encouraged to make use of their religious faith.

Finding meaning and purpose in life and in what has happened. Frankl (1963), the founder of logotherapy, found that discovering meaning and purpose in one's life was helpful in coping with catastrophic experiences such as concentration camps. I have found this to be a very important principle in helping patients who have severe illnesses and suffer serious losses. Many find a purpose in living for their family. Some engage in helping others overcome similar distress, or help others in need. Some lead extremely productive lives despite handicaps. In the acute situation, all these avenues have to be pointed out to the patient. Finding meaning and purpose in what has happened is harder. However, many religions teach this. When patients are religious and take the view that God must have had some purpose in making things happen the way they did, even though the purpose is not always apparent to us mortals, it reduces their distress and guilt.

Changing internal dialogue, relabeling or interpreting the situation, and selective attention. The Greek philosopher Epictetus remarked, "Men are disturbed not by things but by the views which they take of them." (Beck et al. 1979). Cognitive therapists have pointed out that what we pay attention to and what we tell ourselves about a situation affect our mood, that we have control over our emotions, and that we can change our emotions by changing our internal dialogue, i.e., our thinking about the situation (Beck et al. 1979; Meichenbaum 1977). For example, if a patient is saying to himself "Life on hemodialysis is useless. I can not do anything," he can be asked to examine this idea carefully; he may discover that while the hemodialysis does restrict his movement and time schedule, there are a number of things that he can still do to enrich or enjoy his life; in this instance he may change his internal dialogue to, "It is unfortunate that my kidney has failed; but I am happy that at least I have dialysis to help me survive and lead a good life; while there are certain limitations on what I can do, there are still a lot of possibilities for me; let me concentrate my attention on these."

Distraction. This is a type of selective attention, in which one is totally removing attention from a particular idea. Examples are watching television, reading a book, or chatting with others. One problem with the hospital situation is that it is difficult to distract oneself, to keep one's mind occupied much of the time. Occupational therapy is important in the coping process, as being meaningfully and creatively occupied is an effective distractor. Altruistic behaviors (helping others) are also effective distractors (Nadel and Clark 1986). Of course, both of these have the important benefits of promoting self-esteem and sense of purpose, adequacy, utility, and acceptance.

Relaxation techniques. Apart from reducing anxiety and tension, relaxation also improves the patient's sense of being in control.

Grieving. Patients should be encouraged to ventilate their feelings and share their grief with others, especially family members. This is especially important for LRDT rejections. The patient and the family have to be educated about the grieving process and have to be reassured that it is not only "all right" but therapeutic to grieve.

Psychotropic medication. In some situations psychotropic medications may be called for as adjuncts to psychological treatment. If patients develop major depression, they will need antidepressants in addition to psychotherapy. If there is excessive anxiety, they may benefit by use of anxiolytics as adjuncts to psychological intervention.

Obviously the social support system is important for coping. Family support increases the patient's sense of security. Family intervention may be needed to help the family cope with the stress of the patient's illness and to promote optimal interactions between the patient and the family. It is particularly important in the case of LRDT rejection, because of the reverberations in the family, and to mourn the double loss (loss of the kidney by the donor as well as the recipient).

The transplantation and nephrology staff play an important role in the patient's psychosocial adaptation to transplant rejection, by virtue of their special relationship to the patient, their special knowledge, and the amount of time they spend with the patient. Fortunately, these staff members are typically very interested in the patient as a person, know their patients and their families well, have a sound relationship with them, and are caring as well as daring (ready to confront the patient or the family when needed). Staff knowledge of the above-mentioned principles should enable them to help the patient better.

Many patients learn to cope with the loss of a renal transplant, utilizing their own resources and the help of family, friends, and the staff. Psychiatric consultation is usually requested when such an attempt has failed or the patient has become acutely agitated, profoundly depressed, or refuses treatment. The consultant has to assess the situation, including the role of any organic factors (e.g., steroids, antihypertensive medications, infections, uremia, or other metabolic disturbances), competency of the patient, presence of psychosis and suicidal ideation, and the psychodynamics of the situation, including a history of the patient's significant losses and disappointments. This may lead to both organic and psychotherapeutic approaches. The psychotherapy should be primarily supportive (Freyberger 1981), helping the patient ventilate his or her feelings, concerns, conflicts, fears and frustrations, and offering empathy and emotional support. The therapeutic approach should emphasize the here and now and the future, the past being dealt with only to the extent that it is intruding on the present or is immediately relevant to the present. The therapist should be active and should reorient patients from their negative attitudes, encouraging them to be aware of and utilize their strengths and assets (Buchanan 1978). Cognitive behavioral techniques utilizing the coping skills discussed before are useful in this regard. The consultant should also enlist the help of the staff and the family and implement the treatment with their involvement.

CASE ILLUSTRATIONS

Case 1: Diana

Diana was a 35-year-old married woman who received a cadaveric renal transplant after five months of hemodialysis for end-stage renal disease following pyelonephritis. One month after the transplantation, she suddenly developed left hemiparesis and visual impairment due to arterial emboli. When I saw her initially, she was (understandably) very apprehensive about the sudden and progressive loss of various functions. She needed administration of anti-anxiety medication (intramuscular injections of lorazepam) to control her severe anxiety. Subsequently she developed infarction and rejection of the transplanted kidney due to the same embolic process. She became profoundly withdrawn and depressed, did not want to live anymore, and refused all treatment. She saw life as useless, felt that she was a burden on her husband, and felt hopeless. She had no will to live and felt like "ending it all." Quick exploration with her husband in her presence demonstrated to her that she was still very valuable as a person to her husband. She was asked to find a purpose to live for. She decided that her purpose in life was to live for her family. But she was distraught by her neurological dysfunction, felt this would not improve, and was concerned about the quality of her life. I told her that I understood her feelings; that many people have such feelings in the acute stage as it is hard for them to appreciate the potential for rehabilitation and as they have not had sufficient time to develop ways of coping with their losses; that many are later surprised to find how, with medical rehabilitation efforts and with the passage of time, they are able to function much better. I suggested that perhaps she could give herself a few weeks to experience the recovery process. If she still felt like stopping dialysis and other treatment, and giving up, she could do so at that time. She was agreeable to this therapeutic trial. Over the next few weeks there were periods of emotional turbulence, but she responded well to supportive psychotherapy. She also opted for CAPD as she felt that it would give her more independence than hemodialysis would. She engaged energetically in the rehabilitation program, and her mood and functioning improved remarkably within the next few weeks.

Case 2: Joe

Joe was a 35-year-old divorced man with ESRD who became acutely depressed following rejection of his transplanted kidney (donated by his father) three years after the transplantation. He refused hemodialysis as he saw life on hemodialysis as not worth living. He refused to be on hemodialysis even for a period of time while awaiting another (cadaveric) transplantation, as there was no certainty when he would get such a transplant, there was a possibility that he might not get a match, and he was unable to tolerate these uncertainties. He also felt that being on hemodialysis, even for a period of time while awaiting another transplantation, would interfere with his career plans. He agreed to be on hemodialysis temporarily because of pleading from the transplant surgeon, but the staff was uncertain how long he would continue to agree to the dialysis sessions. His family was upset by his desire to discontinue dialysis, and he was angry at his family for not respecting his autonomy. In my encounter with the patient, I let him ventilate his anger and depression, and empathized with him. I told him that I understood how he felt "not in control." I told him that he was competent to refuse dialysis and I respected his autonomy. I pointed out that one could also understand the difficulty his family had in accepting his refusal of dialysis. I offered to meet with him and his family, to facilitate their understanding of his feelings, including his desire for respect for his autonomy, as well as to facilitate his understanding of their feelings. I also told him that perhaps he might consider continuing dialysis for another three or four months to see how things worked out; if he still wanted to discontinue dialysis he could always do so, and we could also discuss this issue with the family. In the family session, other members of the family expressed their recognition of his autonomy to refuse dialysis, even though that decision was painful to them. The patient felt better by the family's show of respect for his autonomy, and decided to continue dialysis for a few months to "see how it worked out," as he now realized that he always had the option to terminate it. During the ensuing weeks, he responded well to psychotherapeutic intervention. Initially he also needed adjunctive use of tranquilizers to help reduce his restless feeling and to help him sleep. Initially the psychotherapy focused on relaxation training, adjusting his goals in life, finding life still meaningful, his self-concept, and changing his internal dialogue and attitudes. Later the therapy also dealt with his conflicted relationship with his father, his rage toward his father for not understanding or respecting his feelings in many matters, and his guilt at the loss of his father's kidney. A couple of conjoint sessions with him and his father were also held, focusing on the father-son interactions and their feelings about each other. The patient's mood improved considerably within a few weeks. As of this writing, the patient has been on hemodialysis for more than two years and has accepted life on hemodialysis.

CONCLUSION

As the above cases illustrate, helping patients cope with the loss of a renal transplant is a challenging experience. One is sharing a deep pain with another person and at the same time helping that person overcome it. This calls for an active, mutifaceted approach, and the results of one's interventions can often be seen immediately or within a short period of time. One is often impressed by the enormous reservoir of inner strength and courage that people have and that can be tapped. The therapist will find it a meaningful and rewarding endeavor.

REFERENCES

Abram, H. S. and D. C. Buchanan. 1976-77. "The Gift of Life: A Review of the Psychological Aspects of Kidney Transplantation. *International Journal of Psychiatry in Medicine* 7: 153-64.

Beck, A. T., A. J. Rush, B. F. Shaw, and G. Emery. 1979. *Cognitive Therapy of Depression*. New York: Guilford.

Beiber, I. 1980. *Cognitive Psychoanalysis*. New York: Jason Aronson.

Buchanan, D. C. 1978. "Psychotherapeutic Intervention in the Kidney Transplant Service." In N.B. Levy, ed. *Psychonephrology 1: Psychological Factors in Hemodialysis and Transplantation*. New York: Plenum, (pp. 265-277).

Castelnuovo-Tedesco, P. 1978. "Transplantation: Psychological Implications of Changes in Body Image." In N.B. Levy, ed. *Psychonephrology 1: Psychological Factors in Hemodialysis and Transplantation*. New York: Plenum, pp. 219-225.

Frankl, V. E. 1963. *Man's Search For Meaning*. New York: Pocket Books.

Freyberger, H. 1983. "The Renal Transplant Patient: Three-stage Model and Psychotherapeutic Strategies." In N.B. Levy, ed. *Psychonephrology 2: Psychological Problems in Kidney Failure and Their Treatment*. New York: Plenum, pp. 259-265.

Gulledge, A. D., C. Buszta, and D. K. Montague. 1983. "Psychosocial Aspects of Renal Transplantation." *Urologic Clinics of North America* 10: 327-335.

Johnson, J. P., C. R. McCauley, and J. B. Copley. 1982. "The Quality of Life of Hemodialysis and Transplant Patients." *Kidney International* 22: 286-291.

Levy, N. B. 1986. "Renal Transplantation and the New Medical Era." In T. N. Wise, ed. *Advances in Psychosomatic Medicine* Vol. 15. Basel: Karger, pp. 167-179.

Meichenbaum, D. 1977. *Cognitive-Behavior Modification*. New York: Plenum.

Monat, A. and R. Lazarus. 1977. 'Stress and Coping: Some Current Issues and Controversies." In A. Monat and R. Lazarus, eds. *Stress and Coping*. New York: Columbia University Press, pp. 1-11.

Nadel, C. and J. J. Clark. 1986. "Psychosocial Adjustment after Renal Retransplants." *General Hospital Psychiatry* 8: 41-48.

Rabin, P. L. 1983. "Psychiatric Aspects of End-Stage Renal Disease: Diagnosis and Management." In W. J. Stone and P. L. Rabin, eds. *End-Stage Renal Disease: An Integrated Approach* New York: Academic Press, pp. 111-147.

Streltzer, J., M. Moe, E. Yanagida, and A. Siemsen. 1983-84. "Coping with Transplant Failure: Grief vs. Denial." *International Journal of Psychiatry in Medicine* 13: 97-106.

Viswanathan, R. 1988. "Helping Patients Cope with Acute Loss of Neuro-muscular Function." *Archives of The Foundation of Thanatology*, 14 (2, Supplement): 20.

Viswanathan, R. and E. K. Kachur. 1986. "Development of Agoraphobia after Surviving Cancer." *General Hospital Psychiatry* 8: 127-132.

Viswanathan, R. and T. Vizner. 1984. "The Experience of Myocardial Infarction as a Threat to One's Personal Adequacy." *General Hospital Psychiatry* 6: 83-89.

III. ETHICAL ISSUES IN TREATMENT OF RENAL DISEASE

Dilemmas in Dialysis: Two Bioethical Case Studies

Daniel J. Klenow

Developments in biomedical technology and life extension have provided a plethora of new social, economic, and ethical challenges and dilemmas. Kidney dialysis, for example, has posed problems of quality of life for some patients and special stresses on medical staff and families (Fox and Swazey 1974; Klenow 1979). The economic costs have not passed without controversy, and a wide variety of ethical issues have surfaced in the literature (O'Brien 1983) and popular press.

This paper seeks to extend and deepen our ethical sensitivity to

Daniel J. Klenow, PhD, is Associate Professor, North Dakota State University, Department of Sociology/Anthropology, Fargo, ND.

Appreciation is expressed to Professors Joy Query and George Youngs, Jr. for providing helpful comments on this paper. Completion of this paper was facilitated through participation in the National Science Foundation/American Academy for the Advancement of Science's Chatauqua Short-Course Program, "Ethical Issues in Death and Dying," conducted by Professor Thomas Beauchamp of Georgetown University.

two types of patient situations in dialysis and transplantation. The dilemmas and communication/interaction problems from these two cases are not unique. Variations of these situations may occur from time to time in most large dialysis/transplant centers. Furthermore, these types of situations are not specific to dialysis and transplantation, but occur, with modifications appropriate to different technologies and treatments, in a wide variety of disease or treatment situations. In short, these cases provide some generic features that can be studied for comparison with other doctor-patient encounters.

METHODS AND PRINCIPLES OF ANALYSIS

The case study material presented in this paper was gathered as part of a larger study of hemodialysis and transplantation. The data were gathered through intensive interviews. The ethical principles of analysis are those frequently cited in the literature on ethical theory (e.g., Beauchamp and Perlin 1978; Childress 1982; Veatch 1976; Thomasma 1983).

BIOETHICAL CASE STUDY 1:
TREATMENT REFUSAL

A 34-year-old male carpenter had been on dialysis for about two years. He seemed to be making a satisfactory adjustment to these treatments and the lifestyle required by them. One afternoon he called the dialysis unit and indicated that he would not be coming in for treatment anymore because his kidneys had been healed. Furthermore, he explained that God had revealed this fact to him in a dream the previous night.

The nephrologist directing the dialysis unit told the patient that he had never heard of such a case. The patient was firm in his belief and the nephrologist closed the conversation by wishing the patient luck and indicating that he would be available if the patient needed help. It is important to know that the patient was supported in his belief by two friends who held similar religious positions. That is to say, they believed in God's direct intervention in everyday life, even when such a view conflicted with well-established medical science.

Within ten days the patient was rushed to the emergency room nearly comatose. He was treated and remained in the hospital for approximately one month. At that time he did not resist treatment, perhaps implicitly acknowledging the need for medical intervention. The residual effects of this episode left him in a wheelchair for over a month. Furthermore, the nephrologists had feared brain damage, but this did not occur.

Ethical Analysis

In this case, at least one critical issue, from an ethical view, concerns the handling of the patient's initial notification that treatment was no longer necessary. The physician was giving priority to the principle of autonomy. Indeed, he indicated that it was not his business to try to change a patient's religious beliefs. The patient, however, was receiving support and social influence from friends of a similar religious orientation. The physician, then, could have argued that he could or should try to exert as much influence as the friends to keep the patient's autonomy potential in balance. The physician might also have tried to expand the patient's conception of the relationship of science and religion by suggesting an alternative interpretation of the dream, namely, that as long as the patient remains on dialysis he is "cured." Many people appreciate the view that dreams, if they mean anything, certainly are not always to be taken literally. In this case, the physician could have presented another symbolic interpretation of the dream. To test his interpretation, the physician could have offered to document the possibility of a cure through a physical examination and appropriate laboratory tests. Such a strategy would allow the physician and patient to explore the meaning of the dream in a way that would, presumably, be as nonthreatening as possible to the patient.

In addition, the physician could have based a course of action that involved trying to change the patient's mind on the principle of beneficence. In short, influencing the patient to continue with treatment would provide a positive good, the good in this case being to preserve the patient's health. This line of ethical analysis is consistent with the position of Thomasma (1983, p. 243), who argues that some models of the physician-patient relationship "fail to provide a place for medicine's beneficence." Thomasma continues (p. 243), "People who are sick need help; their rights to autonomy should not get in the way of their physical needs."

The ethical principle of nonmaleficence can also be brought into the analysis. This principle indicates that an act should do no harm. Clearly, in this case, by structuring his response in such a way as not to influence the patient, a harmful result was ensured. The actual harm in the case included a life-threatening incident that left the patient hospitalized for a month. This is not to say that the physician should attempt to force the patient to take treatment. Indeed, such an act would be legally improbable, based upon established legal precedents. It could be argued from these two ethical principles, however, that the physician should have exerted more influence on the patient.

BIOETHICAL CASE STUDY 2: INCOMPLETE MEDICAL DISCLOSURE

A male dialysis patient, in his mid-twenties, recently had a cadaver kidney transplant that eventually failed. He was returned to home maintenance dialysis after the transplant rejection. This patient is interested in receiving another transplant at some time in the future. Accordingly, he asked his nephrologist if he was back on the transplant list. The physician said yes. The situation, however, is a bit more detailed than the physician's simple affirmation would lead us to believe.

The physician indicated to the researcher that it is highly unlikely that this patient will receive another transplant. The failure of his initial transplant resulted in a complex immunological situation in which the possibility of success for another transplant is extremely low. This patient has been placed in the lowest possible priority position for a transplant and might receive one only if an outstanding match develops. The physician went on to say that he had not given the patient this information because, as he stated, "I have nothing to gain by doing that."

Ethical Analysis

The ethical questions in this case seem to involve the extent of the physician's information exchange with the patient. The full details of the situation are being withheld because the physician feels that he has nothing to gain from such a course of action. Both short-term and long-term utilitarian views can be employed to elucidate this case. From the short-term, utilitarian perspective, it can be surmised that the physician is saving the patient from the pain of knowing that dialysis may well be a lifelong treatment mode. The physician stated that he is leaving the patient with hope regarding the desired transplant option, and this presumably keeps the patient's morale higher than if the truth were known (Klenow 1985).

From the standpoint of long-term utilitarianism, the results of such information withholding may not be so positive. For example, after many years of waiting for a transplant, such a patient may begin to question the nature of his medical condition. The patient will undoubtedly wonder why large numbers of patients have gone on to receive kidney transplants while he continues to wait. He may begin to doubt the information that the physician has given. If, after an extended waiting period, the true nature of this patient's situation is then explained to him, it is very possible that his trust in the medical profession, or at least this physician, will be seriously damaged. There might also be the risk that a negative psychological state may be created if the long-nurtured hope of a transplant is suddenly taken away.

In addition, this case may be examined using Childress' (1982) discussion of modes of nonacquiescence. Passive nonacquiescence is one of these modes. In passive nonacquiescence, a paternalist refuses to carry out the wishes or choices of the patient or to assist the patient in his or her action. Childress states that the disclosure of information in medicine is an affirmative duty and therefore, in this case, passive nonacquiescence typifies the situation. Of course, in this case the physician does not really know what choice the patient would make if given the full details of the medical condition with the contraindications to future transplant attempts.

DISCUSSION

These case studies encourage sensitivity to the complex social, psychological, medical, and ethical dimensions that accompany the use of medical technologies such as hemodialysis and transplantation. Such cases also suggest that health care professionals may be able to expand their range of skills in working with patients by consciously attempting to apply various ethical principles to patient care situations.

The ethical issues raised and principles applied in this paper have been employed in a micro perspective. That is, the ethical analysis has primarily been concerned with the dynamics of the doctor/patient relationship, with no attention directed to the wider context of health care in the United States. Further analysis of such case studies might also apply the principle of distributive justice. In the second case study, for example, the physician might have used distributive justice as an ethical rationale for denying a transplant to the patient, on the grounds that cadaver kidneys are scarce resources that should most appropriately be allocated to those who can benefit from them the most. It is important to realize, however, that the principle of distributive justice cannot be used to justify paternalistic noncommunication with the patient.

REFERENCES

Beauchamp, T. L. and S. Perlin. 1978. *Ethical Issues in Death and Dying.* Englewood Cliffs, NJ: Prentice-Hall.

Childress, J. F. 1982. *Who Should Decide? Paternalism in Health Care.* New York: Oxford University Press.

Fox, R. C. and J. P. Swazey. 1974. *The Courage to Fail: A Social View of Organ Transplants and Dialysis.* Second Edition. Chicago: University of Chicago Press.

Klenow, D. J. 1979. "Staff-Based Ideologies in a Hemodialysis Unit." *Social Science and Medicine.* 13A(6):699-705.

Klenow, D. J. 1985. "Emotion, Work, and Life-Threatening Illness: How Patients Construct Hope." Paper presented at the Midwest Sociological Society Meetings, St. Louis, Missouri.

O'Brien, Mary E. 1983. *The Courage to Survive: The Life Career of the Chronic Dialysis Patient*. New York: Grune and Stratton.

Thomasma, D. C. 1983. "Beyond Medical Paternalism and Patient Autonomy: A Model of Physician Conscience for the Physician-Patient Relationship." *Annals of Internal Medicine*. 98: 243-248.

Veatch, R. M. 1976. *Death, Dying and the Biological Revolution*. New Haven: Yale University Press.

Passions in the Arena

Richard B. Freeman

Should everyone who has a cardiac or pulmonary arrest be resuscitated? Should everyone in need be put on life-support systems? How do we decide whether or not to use high technology medicine for a patient who is about to expire unless some artificial lifesaving device is applied? Do we act if there are only seconds or minutes before life flees from the corporeal body? Does each individual patient *want* to be treated with respirators, pacemakers, dialyzers, etc? What will be the long-term outcome? Will a meaningful life be preserved? Will a patient change his or her mind after experiencing life on artificial support systems? What about the patient who has signed a living will, when the relatives insist that everything be done, or the patient who is still thinking about artificial devices, when time has run out?

When we do not know the whole story, we act. If we don't, a life is lost—forever. We were once taught that, if we do not know what is going on with a patient, the best course is to do nothing. Now, it seems, we do everything.

To gain further insight into the decision-making process, this researcher analyzed experience in a clearly defined situation: institution of dialysis therapy for acute and chronic renal failure. Such therapy is necessary to save a life when the function of the kidneys has deteriorated to a critical point.

Dialysis is a unique therapy. It replaces the function of a vital organ system, the kidneys. It is not an assist device. It differs from respirators and pacemakers that assist the function of the lungs or

Richard B. Freeman, MD, is Chairman, Department of Nephrology, and is Associate Professor of Medicine, University of Rochester School of Medicine, Rochester, NY.

123

the heart. Dialysis can maintain life in the absence of functional parenchymal tissue. Therefore, it is unique and differs from other routine life-support systems.

Patients who received treatment with the artificial kidney for acute and chronic renal failure from 1983 to 1986 were analyzed. Two hundred and twenty-eight patients received therapy in 1983 and 1984, and 482 in the four years from 1983 through 1986. Data is presented on the group analyzed from 1983 and 1984. The groups were divided into six separate categories: acute renal failure following major surgical procedures, acute renal failure due to medical conditions, chronic renal failure patients who were started for the first time on dialysis therapy, and chronic renal failure patients who were admitted for transient illnesses. These groups were compared to patients who had a transplant before 1983 and returned to dialysis because of chronic rejection, and to patients who had new transplants, done during the period of study (Table 1).

The characteristics of the group are presented in Table 2. The age, percentage of males, number of comorbid events, and number of diabetics are listed. In the acute renal failure group, the percentage of males and the mean age of the patients are higher, indicating more vascular disease as a primary cause for their surgical procedures and less tolerance to nephrotoxic agents, increased incidence of hypertensive disease, and other characteristics.

In the chronic renal failure group, the age is slightly lower but the incidence of diabetes is higher as reported by others. The mean age of the transplant group is lower because it includes children and early onset juvenile diabetics.

The number of comorbid conditions was analyzed according to the method of Evans et al. (1985). The numbers of comorbid conditions in ten separate groups were calculated, but the differences in comorbidity were not significantly different between any of the groups. The probable significance of comorbid conditions depends more on severity of a particular condition than on the mere existence of a condition. For example, severe congestive heart failure is more significant than very mild congestive heart failure, although it would be counted as a single comorbid event.

Of interest was the number of DRG categories represented as primary diagnoses. There were 133 categories in which each of the

TABLE 1. Patients Analyzed

	1983-84	1983-86
Acute renal failure (surgical)	36	61
(medical)	59	117
Chronic renal failure - new	42	125
old	32	53
Old failed transplants	10	18
New transplants	49	108
Total	228	482
Total ESRD started in HSA area	200	412

TABLE 2. Characteristics of Group

	AGE	%M	CO-MORBID	DIABETICS	TOTAL PTS
ARF SURGICAL	60.8	81	3.05	3	36
ARF MEDICAL	56.1	69	3.22	5	59
CRF NEW	51.7	52	3.09	9	42
CRF OLD	55.3	41	2.80	10	32
FAILED TRANSPLANTS	37.9	53	3.81	4	10
NEW TRANSPLANTS	38.6	46	2.30	9	49

DRG = 133 CATEGORIES

DRG 315 = 27

DRG 316 = 49

patients who received dialysis fell. Only 27 and 49 patients fell into DRG 315 and 316 respectively, the two categories that are said to cover all of the patients who require dialysis. Clearly, addition of dialysis to DRG categories other than 315 and 316 adds remarkably to the cost and the length of stay of individual patients.

The outcome of the patients in the six groups was divided into those who survived with return of function of their native kidneys, those who survived but continued on dialysis, those who died on dialysis or after acute renal failure had resolved, and patients for whom dialysis therapy was withdrawn (Table 3).

One-third of the acute renal failure patients in the surgical group survived and were discharged from the hospital. For 30 patients, a distinct decision to withdraw dialysis therapy was made.

The variables for each of these patients are numerous. In the first analysis, no definite conclusions could be made regarding the presence of specific disease entities, age, sex, race, or combinations of variables that could predict the outcome.

Table 4 shows the length of stay of each of the groups according to outcome of therapy. Those having the longest stay were the acute renal failure surgical patients who survived their surgical procedure and the accompanying acute renal failure. Of interest is the length of stay of the patients for whom dialysis was withdrawn compared to those who died while on treatment or those who survived on treatment. The key point is that a decision to discontinue treatment did not affect the length of stay of those patients for whom treatment was withdrawn and who subsequently died.

The other major data base available for analysis is the hospital charges for the admission during the event of renal failure that required initiation of dialysis (Table 5). Hospital charges for acute renal failure surgical patients were consistently higher than all other groups, although medical acute renal failure patients had a relatively high charge. There was no difference between hospital charges in patients in whom dialysis therapy was withdrawn compared to those who died on dialysis. A possible conclusion is that efforts to reach a decision to discontinue dialysis did not affect length of stay or hospital charges.

The matter of decision making is key to the compassionate care of patients. It is important to recognize that medicine is not philoso-

TABLE 3. Outcome

	SURVIVED OFF DIALYSIS	SURVIVED ON DIALYSIS	DIED	DIALYSIS WITHDRAWN	TOTAL
ARF SURGICAL	12	2	14	8	36
ARF MEDICAL	16	10	18	15	59
NEW ESRD	0	37	3	2	42
OLD ESRD	0	22	5	5	32
OLD TRANSPLANTS	0	10	0	0	10
NEW TRANSPLANTS	40	7	2	0	49
TOTAL	68	88	42	30	228

TABLE 4. Length of Stay

	SURVIVED OFF DIALYSIS	SURVIVED ON DIALYSIS	DIED	DIALYSIS WITHDRAWN	MEAN
ARF SURGICAL	55.75 (12)	23.50 (2)	25.42 (14)	35.00 (8)	38.14
ARF MEDICAL	30.43 (16)	25.20 (10)	19.08 (18)	25.30 (15)	28.40
NEW ESRD	0	14.57 (37)	36.67 (3)	40.00 (2)	15.21
OLD ESRD	0	12.19 (22)	28.00 (5)	14.60 (5)	13.84
OLD TRANSPLANTS	—	18.27 (10)	—	—	18.27
NEW TRANSPLANTS	19.29 (40)	30.30 (7)	37.00 (2)	—	20.96

TABLE 5. Hospital Charges

	SURVIVED OFF DIALYSIS	SURVIVED ON DIALYSIS	DIED	DIALYSIS WITHDRAWN	TOTAL
ARF SURGICAL	55,330 (12)	22,240 (2)	52,405 (14)	59,136 (6)	36
ARF MEDICAL	25,508 (16)	18,185 (10)	35,342 (18)	27,656 (13)	59
NEW ESRD	0	9,718 (37)	28,921 (3)	25,352 (2)	42
OLD ESRD	0	9,792 (22)	27,788 (5)	24,855 (5)	32
OLD TRANSPLANTS	0	NA (10)	0	0	10
NEW TRANSPLANTS	19,720 (40)	33,410 (7)	49,686 (2)	–	49

phy. It is not ethics, although there is a medical ethic. Medicine is the application of scientific knowledge to set right or to compensate for derangements in the biologic processes of normal human beings. Medicine is also the art of intervention at the correct moment to effect positive changes in deranged biologic mechanisms. The ability to intervene at the proper time demands recognition that a human being must receive psychosocial support and, at times, inspiration in order to overcome adversity. Thus, medicine as a discipline combines special knowledge, timely action, and compassion.

In making decisions regarding application of artificial devices, each patient has the right to participate in the decision-making process. The key concept in this process is to *share* information with the patients and, when appropriate, the family. One does not *tell* patients what will be done, one shares information and relates to them in order to allow them to come to a reasonable decision regarding their long-term care. One always *qualifies* the prognosis. It may not be recognized by the general public that we do not know everything about the biologic processes that function normally in all of us every second of every day. Further, the more we learn about disease processes, the more we know how little we know about so many disorders.

Statements in the literature imply that physicians make errors in diagnoses or judgments. The implication is that mistakes are made, and this certainly is true in some instances. Infinitely more common, however, is the situation where no one knows what the course of a disorder will be, what is appropriate treatment, and what are the mechanisms that have caused this disorder. In other words, we know very little about most pathological disorders and the lack of knowledge makes decision making difficult.

Decisions must be made, however, and the following is offered as a method of reaching a plan for carrying out or withdrawing treatment in an illness where the individual patient's life is threatened.

In individuals who have an unknown diagnosis at the outset or are considered marginal for adapting to chronic maintenance dialysis therapy, it is helpful to agree, at the outset, that there will be a *trial* of therapy. The duration of the trial may be four weeks in patients with acute renal failure, may be a shorter period in patients with chronic renal failure on dialysis who are having severe complications, or may be several months. The proposal of a trial of therapy is presented at the outset of treatment. At the end of the trial, a complete *reevaluation* of the status of the patient is made. The patient is not presented with an ultimatum that a judgment will be made at the end of the trial period; it is simply made clear that a total reevaluation will be made by the medical care team, the patient, and the family, as appropriate.

This method allows patients and families to work through the possibility that existence on artificial life-support systems may be more detrimental than helpful to their life experience. The suffering may be such that it becomes clear to all involved that continuation of therapy is futile.

If it is recognized by the competent patient that there is little chance for rehabilitation, then treatment may be discontinued if the patient agrees. With patients who are mentally incompetent, one must rely on the family to determine whether or not the patient would want to be treated if he or she were competent. In situations where the decision to discontinue therapy is made by the family members, three separate medical opinions should concur that treatment should be discontinued before dialysis is stopped.

If a patient wants to continue therapy, it is his or her right, so far as can be determined under our present social and ethical system. There is a base level of medical therapy that can be offered to all individuals, and at this time dialysis is included in that base.

If the family wants to continue treatment for a patient who is not competent to make his or her own decision, then treatment is continued.

One final principle applied for several patients in this analysis. Any hint of litigation caused the medical professionals to apply every possible means of therapy for those patients.

The principles of decision making, then, are as follows:

1. It is recognized that each individual has multiple known and unknown variables that may affect the course of their disease.
2. Each patient has the freedom of choice to decide whether he or she wishes to have therapy applied or discontinued.
3. For those patients who are competent, each should be treated

as he or she wants to be treated. Each incompetent patient should be treated as he or she would have wanted, so long as such treatment is within reason.

4. Each patient deserves full information, translated from scientific language, so that the patient is totally informed of the medical situation and what the expectations are.

5. Each patient requires time to consider the alternatives, and the medical professionals must be patient and compassionate in this decision making.

6. The basic principle of medicine has not changed. Each patient deserves to be healed if possible, kept comfortable if they cannot be healed, and spared from harm.

There is a certain passion that pervades the center of the decision-making arena. This emotion certainly occurs in the majority of patients and patient families. It affects medical professionals because we, too, are involved in mankind. Attempts to describe this passion to those outside the center of the arena causes bewilderment, anxiety, or anger. Those who have never been directly responsible for moderating discussions on such decisions find difficulty in understanding this emotion. It is unusual that individuals outside of the medical profession understand the limitations of our science and our art. Therefore, it is those individuals in the center of the arena that should set the standards for rational, compassionate, and reasonable decision making. We share information, we qualify the prognosis, we tell the truth. No one has all the answers. We moderate the discussions rather than directing them, so that the central character in the drama can reach the best possible decision.

Nature provides many challenges to us all. When we contend with nature for our own gain, we have interfered unjustly. When we strive to enhance nature, we act in beneficence for all of humanity.

REFERENCE

Evans, R. G., D. L. Manninen, L. P. Garrison, L. G. Hart, C. R. Blagg, R. A. Gutman, A. R. Hull, and E. G. Lowrie. 1985. "The Quality of Life of Patients with End-Stage Renal Disease." *New England Journal of Medicine* 312:553-559.

Kidney Transplants:
A Jewish Perspective

Shelley M. Buxbaum

Judaism regards human life as being of infinite value. The commandment to save a life overrides all others; all required obligations and restrictions with reference to Sabbath observance are lifted whenever there is a possibility of saving a life (Yoma 85b). Furthermore, it is pointed out that he who is responsible for saving one life is considered as one who has saved the entire world. Jewish law regards the physician as being a partner with God in acting on behalf of his fellow men. A physician is legally obligated to render medical care not only in life-threatening situations but also as is required to alleviate pain or to preserve physical well-being.

The obligation to heal is established in the Torah. Leviticus 19:16 states, "Nor shall you stand idly by the blood of your fellow." In verse 18 of the same chapter we find, "And you shall love your neighbor as yourself." And in Deuteronomy 22:2 we read, "and you shall restore it [health] to him." From these verses we learn that an authorized physician is thereby granted permission to heal his fellow human beings.

This principle is further amplified in the Talmud. Pesachim 25a teaches, "We may use any material for healing except that which is connected with idolatry, immorality, and bloodshed." Maimonides, a twelfth-century physician and philospher, advises the seriously ill patient to obey his physician even when informed that he can be cured by a certain object which may be forbidden by law. In his major work, *Guide to the Perplexed*, Maimonides suggests the following guidelines for a physician to follow as he considers his op-

---

Shelley M. Buxbaum is a doctoral candidate at the Jewish Theological Seminary of America, New York, NY.

tions for treatment: (1) use anything which has been proven effective in practice even though it is not understood how it operates and why; (2) make a decision that follows as a rational deduction from generally accepted physical theory; and (3) always seek advice and opinion from peer physicians.

When we consider the monumental strides achieved in medical science, it becomes clear that the ancient texts can only provide us with a hint as to how to face the options and alternatives that are now available. Therefore, it has become the responsibility of recognized rabbis to address themselves to these new options and alternatives as they advise their congregants on how to make decisions for treatment that will be commensurate with Jewish law. The genre of Responsa Literature provides the mechanisms by which these decisions can be discussed.

The consensus among contemporary rabbis is that whenever there is a possibility, however remote, of improving a patient's chances of recovery, he is to be considered as having nothing to lose. This prospect of short-term benefit may be risked to achieve any prolongation of life. We may conclude from this decision that if organ transplantation is performed to cure or alleviate a life-threatening condition, then it is permissible by Jewish law.

Let us now turn our attention to the question at hand, namely, a patient experiencing renal failure. Dr. Fred Rosner (Professor of Medicine, State University of New York at Stony Brook, and recognized scholar of Jewish law) has stated, "A kidney transplant is only undertaken when both kidneys of the recipient are so diseased that life cannot continue without the removal of the body's waste products that accumulate in the blood" (1983, p. 356). However, he hastens to point out that "it is categorically prohibited to prepare a critically ill donor for transplantation surgery if this preparation in any way hastens his death" (p. 356).

Having established the validity of the transplant procedure, Rosner goes on to say that, if one death has occurred, it is permissible to delay burial and remove the corpse's kidneys because of the consideration of saving another life.

With regard to living donors, the rabbis have addressed themselves to the following questions: (1) Who may donate a kidney? (2) Is a donor permitted to subject himself to danger in order to save another life? (3) How does one decide who is to receive the available kidney? For answers we again turn to Responsa Literature. According to Sir Immanuel Jakobovits, Chief Rabbi of England, a donor may endanger his own life or health to supply a spare organ to a recipient whose life would thereby be saved (Federation of Jewish Philanthropies of New York 1984). According to Rabbi Eliezer Waldenberg of Jerusalem's Shaarey Zedek Hospital, "Kidney transplants from a live donor are only permissible if a group of trustworthy physicians testifies that there is no danger to the life of the donor and if the donor is not coerced into consenting to the procedure" (1980). Most rabbinical authorities agree with these two opinions. While one is not obligated to donate an organ for transplantation, one who does so in order to save the life of another has clearly performed an act of loving kindness.

Conservative Rabbis belonging to the Rabbinical Assembly have suggested the following resolution at a recent convention:

> Whereas Judaism places the highest value on human life; and
>
> Whereas we now have new and wonderful opportunities for saving lives and improving the quality of life through the transplantation of organs; and
>
> Whereas there is a great shortage of organs available for transplant, with long waiting lists of patients desperate for a chance at life, and dying still waiting for a heart, a kidney or other organ; and
>
> Whereas there are tremendous expenses involved in these procedures, far beyond the reach of most individuals and families;
>
> Therefore, be it resolved that the Rabbinical Assembly support the process of organ transplantation and the donation of organs according to halakhah towards that end. We call upon all persons to sign and carry organ donor cards. We call upon families who have suffered the loss of a loved one to allow their tragedy to become an opportunity for life for another human being, through the donation of the deceased's organs for transplant; and
>
> Be it further resolved that we petition both state and federal

governments to help fund the expensive procedure of organ transplantation so that no one will die simply for lack of funds.

Adoption of this resolution is now subject to review by the Committee on Jewish Law and Standards.

While agreeing in principle to the permissibility of live donors for organ transplants, Rabbi David Bleich, a noted authority on Jewish bioethics, questions the validity of the Uniform Donor Act for Jews. He takes exception to the "blanket authorization" on the donor card, which states that "body parts may be used for purposes of therapy, medical research, or education." In addition to the unrestricted use of body parts, Rabbi Bleich points out that there is no provision for the ultimate return of the organ for burial, which is a requirement of Jewish law.

Rabbi Solomon Freehof, representing the Reform Movement, concurs with the above-stated opinions. He bases his decision on the Maimonidean guidelines we discussed above.

Turning our attention to the recipient, we find the following definition, which the rabbis have accepted. A recipient is one who is in a clear and present danger and who is capable of benefiting directly from the transplant procedure. However, since the demand far outweighs the supply, allocation must be done by a fair, arbitrary, and random selection among those who possess therapeutic hope.

REFERENCES

Federation of Jewish Philanthropies. 1984. *The Compendium on Medical Ethics* (6th ed.)

Rosner, F. 1983. "Organ Transplantation in Jewish Law." In F. Rosner and J. D. Bleich, eds. *Jewish Bioethics*. New York: Hebrew Publishing Co.

Waldenberg, E. 1980. *Tzitz Eliezer* Vol. IX, Sect. 44. In A. Steinberg, ed. *Jewish Medical Law*, D. Simons, trans. Jerusalem: Gefen Publishing.

Promoting Organ Donation Among Memorial Society Members

Katherine Diaz-Knauf
Howard Schutz
Robert Sommer

Recent years have seen dramatic changes in the treatment of terminal diseases of the kidney, liver, heart, lungs, and other organs. Previously, people suffering from diseases of these organs generally died, but now the successful transplantation of organs offers a lifesaving alternative. As valuable as these techniques are, their use has been seriously limited by the availability of suitable organs. More than a third of patients on a waiting list for liver transplants and one-half of those waiting for a heart transplant die before a donor organ can be found (Ringe et al. 1985; Robertson 1987). An organ shortage also extends the length of time that individuals with life-threatening illnesses must endure their severe medical condition. The waiting time for transplanted livers may be as long as two years (Gold et al. 1986). The psychological costs to patients and their families of a prolonged wait for a donor organ include economic difficulties created by extended hospitalization, disruption of the lives of family members, lack of mobility, pervasive fear that the patient will die before a donor organ is found, and feelings of depression and helplessness (Perkins 1987). The scarcity of donor

Katherine Diaz-Knauf, MPA, is Staff Research Associate, Department of Consumer Sciences, and Howard Schutz, PhD, is Professor of Consumer Sciences, University of California at Davis, Davis, CA. Robert Sommer, PhD, is Professor of Psychology, and is Director of The Center for Consumer Research, University of California at Davis, Davis, CA.

The assistance of R. Almeida, B. Flory, and L. Servus is gratefully acknowledged.

organs also creates ethical dilemmas as to who should have the few that become available. Ironically, as the success rate of transplant procedures continues to increase, the shortfall of donatable organs becomes more severe.

Three major factors needed to increase supply are: (1) an adequate supply of donors, (2) the willingness of relatives to accede to a donation, and (3) the efficient location of donors, especially for small hospitals and those in rural areas. In 1986, it was estimated that as many as 27,500 individuals were declared brain-dead, thus becoming potential donors, but fewer than 20 percent of this group became the source of transplant organs.

Obtaining consent from the family to procure organs is often considered to be the most critical step (Iglehart 1983; Overcast et al. 1984). Professional education can remedy problems in identifying appropriate donors and initiating a request to the family, but failure to obtain family consent occurs in approximately half of all requests (Sales and Burrows 1986). This suggests the value of educational programs directed specifically to families rather than to individuals. Educational campaigns are likely to come up against the various death-related taboos and fears in American society. This is not a topic that most people, particularly those who are young and healthy, want to hear or think about. Some of the unwillingness of families to authorize donation stems from unarticulated fears and perceived risks of premature organ removal and a lack of understanding about the nature of brain death (Shanteau 1986).

The need for greater family involvement suggested the value of working with memorial societies in promoting organ donation. Since its inception a half-century ago, the memorial society movement has become a vanguard in campaigns for preplanning. There are 200 memorial societies operating in North America, with a total membership of a million households. These nonprofit, nonsectarian volunteer organizations are dedicated to education and consumer protection in all death-related activities. They have not been particularly active in organ donation and procurement. The advantages of greater involvement of memorial societies in organ donation appeals are as follows:

1. They are organizations specifically formed around death-related activities and committed to public discussion and awareness. The desensitization necessary to broach this topic in most other groups would be largely unnecessary.
2. The societies already promote donation of bodies to medical schools as one alternative. To broaden this concept to vital organ donation seems a feasible and realizable objective.
3. Memorial societies view organ donation as a relevant area in their own agendas.
4. Societies are primarily educational in nature; their activities include maintaining lists and records, distributing educational materials and permission forms, and publishing a newsletter. All these activities would be useful in an organ donation campaign.
5. Membership consists primarily of older, well-educated men and women, established in the community, including a high proportion of retired educators (Sommer, Hess, and Nelson 1985). These conditions are suited to members becoming a vanguard in promoting organ donation in their own families and in the larger community.
6. Membership is typically by household or family. Educational programs can therefore be directed at the family unit. Treating the decision as a family matter should make it easier to get consensus and thereby obtain permission at the appointed time.
7. There is a widespread perception among the memorial society leadership that the organizations are experiencing a loss of identity and purpose. Many of the original objectives, such as promotion of cremation and simple, low-cost funerals, are being offered by direct disposition firms. There is a feeling that the organizations need new goals and objectives that might logically include organ donation as a socially important, death-related activity.

The present study explores the potential for greater involvement of memorial society members in vital organ procurement through public education and donation appeals. From a strategic standpoint in changing public attitudes, there is value in targeting, not those who care little about an issue, but those who have already expressed an interest that can be converted into action. The study also explores the relative value for this target audience of three different types of appeals identified in the organ donation literature as likely to promote attitude change. The *rational appeal* centers on objective needs related to the shortage of donor organs, the benefits of transplantation, statistics on positive outcomes, and savings to society in hospital costs. The *emotional appeal* is intended to arouse sympathy by particularizing appeals around specific individuals who can be helped. *Altruistic appeals* demonstrate concern for the welfare of others, fulfillment of a higher purpose, and service to the community.

We wanted to see if there might be differential impact among the three types of appeals for memorial society members. This would be measured in increased discussion of donation with family members and willingness to return a signed pledge card.

MATERIALS

Appeal Brochures

From the technical literature on organ donation appeals and the materials used by organ donation agencies across the country, three types of appeals were identified: *rational* (emphasizing the facts about donation needs), *emotional* (emphasizing the personal hardship and benefits in donation), and *altruistic* (emphasizing the gift aspects of donation). Three brochures representing these three appeals were developed and pretested for appropriateness in a class of university students.

General Design of the Study

The first phase of the study involved a test of the three appeals using a postcard on which the respondent indicated a willingness to sign a donation card. Following this, a mail survey was conducted to test the effectiveness of the three appeals on a variety of attitudinal measures.

METHOD

Phase I: Postcard Response to Appeals

A mail survey of 2,000 members of the Sacramento Valley Memorial Society (SVMS) was conducted using the society's membership list. In addition, 200 Sacramento area residents were surveyed using the Sacramento area telephone directory as the sampling frame. A systematic random sampling procedure was employed during November/December 1987. SVMS members were randomly assigned to one of the appeal groups or a control group. A second control group was made up of Sacramento area residents (nonmembers). Individuals in the two control groups received a letter, a uniform organ donor card, and a response card. SVMS members assigned to one of the three appeal groups received a letter and brochure tailored for the specific type of appeal, a uniform donor card, and a response card. Five hundred and eighty responses were received (28 percent of all deliverable response forms). Four response forms arrived too late to be included in the tabulations.

Cross-tabulation of week of return by type of appeal did not indicate any statistically significant monotonic trend differences over time — evidence that there is minimal nonresponder bias.

Phase II:
Questionnaire Response to Appeals

Two weeks after the initial survey, the 1,800 members of the SVMS sample were sent a letter and a questionnaire on the topic of organ donation. Thirty-seven percent of 1,699 delivered questionnaires were completed and returned. The four-page questionnaire required approximately 15 minutes to complete. Cross-tabulation of week of return by type of appeal did not indicate any statistically significant monotonic trend differences over time — evidence that there is minimal nonresponder bias.

Respondents were asked to assess the effectiveness of the brochures, their knowledge and attitudes concerning organ and tissue transplantation, amount of discussion on these topics with others, attitudes about donation (of organ and tissue), willingness to donate for transplantation to family and nonfamily members, and demographic characteristics.

RESULTS

Phase I: Postcard Response to Appeals

Overall, 34.1 percent of the memorial society members had previously signed a pledge card. These results are considerably higher than the 19.2 percent reported in a nationwide survey among the general public (Manninen and Evans 1985), demonstrating the high level of interest among this group in the topic.

Of the 382 individuals who responded that they had not previously signed a pledge card, 136 (35.6 percent) checked that they had signed our pledge card. Although there are no significant differences among the appeal groups, results of our cross-tabulations show a trend for the *altruistic* appeal to be more effective — 42.9 percent versus 37.4 percent and 29.7 percent for the *emotional* and *rational* appeal, respectively. The nonmember control group was considerably lower in the number of signed pledges, 17.6 percent versus 34.3 percent for members, although not statistically significant. Pledge discussion results for those not previously signing a pledge card show that overall 147 (38.5 percent) discussed their pledge. For the *altruistic* appeal group (those who did not check having previously signed a pledge card), 93.2 percent reported discussing their pledge with family, 4.8 percent with other family, and 2.1 percent with nonfamily. These differences were not statistically significant.

Of those individuals who had previously signed a pledge card or the enclosed donor card, 265 (45.7 percent) reported having discussed their pledge. Of this number, the vast majority (91.7 percent) had discussed the pledge with their immediate family, 5.3 percent with other family members, and 3 percent with nonfamily members. Two hundred twenty-six society members (39 percent) indicated that they did not want to make a pledge at this time.

Phase II:
Characteristics of the Respondents

The distribution of respondents by sex, age, ethnicity, education, and income is presented in Table 1. Of 625 respondents, 341 (54.7 percent) were male. Four hundred and seventy (75.8 percent) were 60 years old or older. Ninety-eight percent were Caucasian. Three hundred and seventy-six (61 percent) had a college degree. Forty-

TABLE 1: Demographic characteristics of sample of Sacramento Valley Memorial society members.

	n	%
SEX:		
Male	341	54.7
Female	282	45.3
	623	
AGE:		
20-29	1	.2
30-39	12	1.9
40-49	35	5.6
50-59	102	16.5
60-69	209	33.7
70-79	194	31.3
80+	67	10.8
	620	
ETHNICITY:		
White-Caucasian	611	98.2
Other	11	1.8
	622	
EDUCATION:		
Less than high school graduate	36	5.9
High school graduate	57	9.3
Some college	147	23.9
College graduate and more	376	61.0
	616	
INCOME:		
< $10,000	57	9.7
10,000-19,999	121	20.5
20,000-29,999	95	16.1
30,000-39,999	115	19.5
40,000-49,999	66	11.2
50,000+	135	22.9
	589	

seven percent of the members reported earnings of $20,000 to $49,999, and 22.9 percent reported earnings over $50,000. These results are similar to those reported in an earlier study of California memorial society members (Sommer, Hess, and Nelson 1985).

The Brochures

Eighty percent of the sample recalled receiving the brochure (see Table 2); 58.5 percent said they "read it closely" and 33.5 percent "read it some," while 7.9 percent said they "did not read" the brochure. The pamphlet was seen as informative by 93 percent of the respondents, easy to understand by 92 percent, easy to read by 86 percent, and factual by 83 percent. Only 32 percent found the brochure to contain new knowledge, compared with 42 percent considering it "old knowledge." There was significantly higher perception of new knowledge in the *altruistic* and *rational* appeals than with the *emotional* appeals ($X^2 = 6.6$. s.d. $= 2$, p $< .05$).

Transplantation Information

There were several general information questions pertaining to transplantation. The overwhelming majority of respondents (87.5 percent) indicated that in terms of priorities for medical research, donation was "important" or "very important." Fifty-seven per-

TABLE 2: SVMS members' ratings of the effectiveness of the brochures.

ATTRIBUTES*	EMOTIONAL		RATIONAL		ALTRUISTIC	
	n	%	n	%	n	%
Informative	79	33.9	85	36.5	69	29.6
Factual	53	32.9	57	35.4	51	31.7
New knowledge	14	26.4	17	32.1	22	41.5
Easy to read	53	31.4	59	34.9	57	33.7
Easy to understand	65	30.7	68	32.1	79	37.3

*The percentage represents those individuals rating in the highest category for each attribute.

cent felt that there was a "very serious shortage" of organs and tissues available for donation, while 21.8 percent said there was "some shortage." When asked who should be primarily responsible for payment for transplantation procedures, 42.4 percent said "private insurance," 20.9 percent "government agency," 19.1 percent "other," and 17.5 percent "individual." Overall, there were no significant differences between appeal groups.

Discussion with Family and Nonfamily Members

SVMS members were asked whether they had ever discussed donation with family and nonfamily members prior to receiving the materials we sent. The overwhelming majority (72.8 percent) of respondents indicated that they had discussed this issue with family members prior to receiving the brochure. The majority (52.7 percent) indicated they had also discussed donation issues with nonfamily members. Almost half (49 percent) had discussed donation issues with family members after receiving the brochure, and of this number 77 percent indicated that their family members agreed to the importance of this issue relative to other medical issues that face our society today. There were no significant differences noted among the appeal groups.

Attitudes Toward Donation

Respondents were asked whether they had major reservations about being donors themselves. The majority (73.5 percent) did not have any major reservations about being a donor, 21.9 percent said "yes," while 4.6 percent "didn't know." Age was the most common reason cited by the respondents who said they had reservations about being a donor. Other reasons were "general uneasiness" (13.8 percent), "generally poor health" (10.6 percent), while 15.4 percent listed "other" and did not elaborate. Respondents were asked what they perceive is the major value in people donating organs or tissue. Forty-five percent said "helping fellow human being," 21.8 percent said it "saves lives," and 16.7 percent answered "other" without elaboration. There were no significant differences noted among the appeal groups.

Willingness to Donate

SVMS members were asked a series of questions regarding their willingness to donate to family and nonfamily members. The majority (74.9%) said "yes" they would be willing to donate a kidney to a family member, compared to 62.4 percent to a nonfamily member. There were no significant differences among the appeal groups.

Only four percent of the respondents indicated that a family member had previously donated. Of those, donations included "cornea" 34.8 percent, "sclera-opaque outer coat of eyeball" 21.7 percent, "kidney" and "entire body" 17.4 percent, and "other" 8.7 percent.

Members were asked if up to the time they received the pamphlet they had completed and signed a uniform donor card. Forty-six percent of the respondents said "yes," 41.5 percent said "no," and 2.4 percent "didn't know." The overwhelming majority (85.7 percent) had signed the card supplied by the state Department of Motor Vehicles. Sixty-eight percent had pledged "any needed organs and/ or tissues" and 24.1 percent their "entire body." Fifty-seven percent said "yes" they had informed members of their family of their willingness to be an organ and/or tissue donor, and instructed them to notify the attending physician of their wishes, 40.7 percent said "no," and 2.7 percent said they "didn't know." There were no significant differences noted among appeal groups.

DISCUSSION

The results from Phase I dramatically illustrate the higher level of interest in the organ donation area for members of a memorial society as compared to the general population. This is shown both by a higher response rate for the three appeal groups, as well as the memorial society control group, as compared to the general population control group in the Sacramento area. In addition, a high level of pledges in the memorial society groups both before and after our request as compared to the general population underscores this difference in attitude. As pointed out in the results, the 34.1 percent of SVMS members who had previously signed a card is considerably higher than the approximately 19 percent that has been reported in nationwide studies.

The lack of differentiation among the three types of appeals, *altruistic*, *rational*, and *emotional*, is perhaps not surprising, in view of the preexisting high level of interest in the topic among all groups who received the brochure. Our belief that memorial society members would discuss the issue with their families is borne out by the almost three-quarters of the respondents who had discussed the issue with their families prior to receiving the brochure and the half again who had discussed it after receiving the brochure. Almost three-quarters indicated that they did not have any major reservations about being a donor. All these responses demonstrate the positive outlook of memorial society members toward organ donation.

Since the societies already conduct outreach programs on death-related issues, there would appear to be value in developing organ donation appeals specifically for these groups. While the membership largely represents older, well-educated, and somewhat affluent individuals, they can be a vanguard within the general population, and their attitudes can certainly influence their children and grandchildren on organ donation and other death-related issues. On a more theoretical basis, these results lead to the conclusion that a more rational, healthy attitude toward death and dying can be associated with values that are not only beneficial to the individual but to society as a whole.

REFERENCES

Gold, L. M., B. S. Kirkpatrick, F. J. Fricker, and B. J. Ziteli. 1986. "Psychosocial Issues in Pediatric Organ Transplantation: The Parents' Perspective." *Pediatrics* 77:738-744.

Iglehart, J. K. 1983. "Transplantation: The Problem of Limited Resources." *New England Journal of Medicine* 309:123-128.

Overcast, T. D., R. W. Evans, L. E. Bowen, M. M. Hoc, and C. L. Livak. 1984. "Problems in the Identification of Potential Organ Donors." *Journal of the American Medical Association* 251(12):1559-1562.

Perkins, K. A. 1987. "The Shortage of Cadaver Donor Organs for Transplantation." *American Psychologist* 41:921-930.

Ringe, B., P. Neuhaus, R. Pichlmayr, and B. Heigel. 1985. "Aims and Practical Application of a Multi-procurement Protocol." *Langenbecks Archives Chirurgie* 365:47-55.

Robertson, J. A. 1987. "Supply and Distribution of Hearts for Transplantation: Legal, Ethical, and Policy Issues." *Circulation* 75:77-87.

Sales, C. M. and L. Burrows. 1986. "Cadaveric Organ Transplantation Procurement: An Investigation of the Source of Kidney Shortages." *Transplantation Proceedings* 18:416-418.

Shanteau, J. 1986. "Psychological Research on Organ Donation, Advances in Health Care Research." *Proceedings of American Association for Advances in Health Care Research*, pp. 89-90.

Sommer, R., K. Hess, and S. Nelson. 1985. "Funeral Co-op Members' Characteristics and Motives." *Sociological Perspectives* 28(4):487-500.

IV. STAFF/PATIENT PERSPECTIVES IN CARE OF RENAL DISEASE

Dialysis Staff Attitudes Toward Providing End-Stage Care

Timothy E. Tennyson
James H. Jennison
N. D. Vaziri

While we were involved in research on a dialysis unit several years ago, the staff mentioned to us that working in chronic hemodialysis was different from working in other hospital settings. We asked what was unique about a hemodialysis unit. Responses included that there were fewer acute crises than in other hospital units, that there were no night hours, and that staff got to know patients very well. A family environment was described.

One of the patients was found dead in her apartment during the time we worked on the study. There had been no physical indica-

Timothy E. Tennyson, PhD, is in private practice (psychology), South Coast Psychological Services, Irvine, CA. James H. Jennison, PhD, is affiliated with the Department of Physical Medicine and Rehabilitation, School of Medicine, University of California (Irvine), Orange, CA. N.D. Vaziri, MD, is Vice Chair and Chief, Nephrology Division, University of California, Irvine Medical Center, Irvine, CA.

151

tions of her impending death in the days previous. Several of the staff approached us and told us that a patient's death was the most difficult part of working on a dialysis unit. They asked for an inservice presentation on how to deal with such an occurrence.

Descriptions of the dialysis unit as a unique place to work are common among nursing staff. Patients are chronically dependent on the dialysis treatment for their physical survival. Their reactions to this reality vary according to demographic, physical, personal, and environmental factors. One of the environmental factors they encounter is the attitude of the staff members (McCarron 1973). Dialysis staff also find themselves acting a role in relation to these patients that is determined by both the dialysis setting and their own attitudes toward health care and death. The death of a patient has a profound effect on staff in this setting.

This paper assumes that staff attitudes influence the clinical relationship on the dialysis unit (Stein 1985). It attempts to illuminate the subjective interaction between staff and patient that is determined by the interactive style and attitudes of a staff member. Knowledge about patients' process and perspective related to their health and death forms only a part of our understanding of issues related to their treatment. Knowledge about how we relate to those same concepts is another part (Stein 1979). We investigated the way dialysis staff persons describe their attitudes to health and death, how those attitudes relate to each other, as well as how a personality type may influence those issues. We also made a preliminary attempt to define what is unique about dialysis staff attitudes to life, health, and death. The constructs used to define each area are reflected by the measure utilized.

METHODS

Twenty dialysis staff participated in this preliminary study. Attitude toward death was measured by the Templer Death Anxiety Scale (TDAS) (Templer 1970). This scale is designed to be a short measure of "death anxiety." The Health Locus of Control scale (HLOC) was used to determine where a person placed responsibility for his or her own health. Finally, the Myers-Briggs Personality

Type Indicator (MBTI) was used to provide a description of a person's orientation to life. We were interested in the power of these measures to describe the dialysis staff member.

Templer Death Anxiety Scale

The Templer Death Anxiety Scale is a 15-item, true-false scale designed to measure death anxiety. Although other measures have been suggested, this scale is the most commonly held standard in the measurement of the death anxiety construct. TDAS norms were established using both healthy subjects and patients diagnosed as psychotic, neurotic, and having personality disorders (Templer 1970).

Death Anxiety

The construct of death anxiety has been much studied in relation to personality, environmental, and psychopathological factors in a variety of populations. Some have argued that death anxiety represents a "state" phenomenon, but a recent study concluded that evidence suggests it is a "trait" (Pettigrew and Dawson 1979). The literature does not support any clear relationship between death anxiety and occupational choice (Lattanner and Hayslip 1984). We were interested to see whether personal attitudes and beliefs about one's own health may correlate with death anxiety measures within a specific occupational group, especially one dealing with terminal patients.

Health Locus of Control Scale

The Health Locus of Control Scale (HLOC) was designed by Wallston and her colleagues (1976) as a means of exploring the relationship of locus of control to health behaviors. Based on the more generalized construct of Rotter's (1966) Internal-External Locus of Control Scale, they developed an 11-item scale using a six-point, Likert-type format for responses. The sum of scores is then interpreted as an indication of internal or external locus of control when it comes to matters of health or illness. Individuals with high scores are seen as "health externals" and are presumed to expect that factors such as luck, chance, or powerful others are the determinants of their state of health.

The HLOC gives a measure of "personalized" perspective on one's own state of health which may, in part, be reflected in the level of death anxiety. A previous study of HLC and death anxiety (Tolor 1978) found no relationship. Another study of Rotter's I-E (O'Dowd 1984-85) found more acceptance of immortality concepts among internals, but correlation with death anxiety did not reach significance. Both the Templer and HLOC scales were administered in this study in order to further explore any possible relationship. The relationship of TDAS and HLOC with the MBTI was also investigated.

Myers-Briggs Type Indicator

The Myers-Briggs Type Indicator (MBTI) is a forced-choice, self-report inventory that attempts to describe individuals according to an adaptation of Carl Jung's theory of conscious psychological type (Myers 1962). It assumes behavior is consistently based on a person's style of interaction with his or her world (Jung 1923). The MBTI classifies by four dichotomous dimensions. The first dimension is a general attitude toward the world. An attitude directed outward to other persons and objects is described as extroverted (E). An attitude focused on internal representations of events is called introverted (I). The E-I dimension does not measure gregariousness, but whether a person relies on internal or external constructs in their interaction with their world.

The second dimension of the MBTI defines perception. Sensing (S) refers to attending to actual sensory realities; paying attention to facts and details. Intuition (N), on the other hand, is a more global attention to possibilities and insight based on the data the person receives. The (S) personality type attends to the trees at the expense of the forest while the (N) attends to the forest at the expense of the trees.

The third dimension defines whether the person uses primarily thinking (T) or feeling (F) in making judgments. Thinking refers to a reliance on reasoning and logic while feeling refers to a reliance on more subjective personal impressions compared on a value basis.

The final dimension is based on how a person tends to make decisions. A willingness to make quick decisive conclusions is defined as judging (J). A preference to hold off decisions while "gathering more data" is defined as perceiving (P) (Willis 1982).

Each dimension is labeled by an individual's dominant process. The dominant process is the one on which the person relies the most. Combinations of the four dimensions result in one of sixteen possible personality types. The four letters "ISFJ," for example, define a personality type belonging to an individual whose attention and energy is directed to internal representations of events (I); who notices facts and details (S); who uses a subjective, feeling style to make judgments (F); and who is willing to make quick, conclusive decisions (J) (Myers 1962; Willis 1982).

HYPOTHESES

In addition to constructing a definition of the average attitudes and personality of a dialysis staff person, we predicted that persons who demonstrated an internal locus of control related to their own health issues would show lower death anxiety than those who placed the control of their health in externals. High scores on the TDAS would be matched by low scores on the HLOC.

We predicted that MTBI factors introversion (I) vs. extroversion (E) would correlate with both TDAS and HLOC scores. Here we were interested in the relationship between the constructs of "Introversion/Extroversion" and "death anxiety" as well as "locus of control."

Predicted also was that the score of the TDAS would correlate with answers to the question "Has the death of a patient affected you more than the death of a relative," and a self-rating (1 to 10) of the effect a patient's death has had on the staff member. The idea behind the inclusion of these questions was that a patient's death is the most probable event to elicit death anxiety in a dialysis setting.

RESULTS

No significant relationship between the TDAS, HLOC, and MBTI was noted.

TDAS

The mean score on the TDAS was 4.6, with all scores within normal limits.

HLOC

The mean score on the HLOC was 33, also within normal limits.

MBTI

Registered nurses gave significantly more extroverted responses than technicians (p = .03).

A "mean profile" was constructed by tabulating the total "continuous scores" of the staff subjects described by the MBTI manual (Myers 1977). The resulting "ISFJ" personality type is described below.

ISFJ

The ISFJ temperament is found in only six out of every one hundred people. The least hedonistic of the sixteen personality types, they are described as being dependable, devoted, traditional, and responsible. They are able to work long and hard providing routine services. With a primary desire to care for individuals, they relate best to people who need them. ISFJs relate to persons rather than to institutions. They expect others, including the boss, to follow procedures and are distressed when people do not behave as they are supposed to behave. Speculation or philosophical concerns do not intrigue ISFJs; they are most comfortable with immediate, "down-to-earth" concerns (Keirsey 1984).

While being dependable, the ISFJ may be fascinated by the irresponsible. Many marry alcoholics and play a rescue-rejection game without end. When female, they often act out a "double standard," being resigned to the "waywardness" of men while expecting women to respect time-honored traditions. Stress is internalized by this personality type into fatigue and muscle tension.

At work the ISFJ seems to feel responsible to see that everyone carries out established procedures. They abhor the squandering of resources. Instead they value saving resources to prepare for emergencies. This personality type experiences discomfort when placed in positions of authority. When promoted they find themselves trying to do everything rather than insisting that others do their jobs.

ISFJs are frequently taken for granted. They do not demand overt recognition for their contributions. Easily misunderstood and undervalued, they often hide their hurt and suffering. This can turn to hidden resentment and covert attempts to regain control of their environment (Keirsey 1984).

CONCLUSION

TDAS and HLOC

The TDAS and HLOC showed no differences among staff members. A larger sample of staff may be required. The power of both measures to discriminate among healthy subjects is questioned. Both measure only the surface dynamics of a person's cognitive style. Both are an indicator of the person's "state" of death anxiety and locus of control (Pettigrew 1979). Traditional, conforming responses to the statements on both scales were demonstrated. Underlying personality traits are not addressed. Both measures may be summarized by simple one-sentence questions about the person's present perspective. The statement, "I am very much afraid to die" is as valid and reliable as the whole TDAS (Holmes 1980). The statement, "It is up to me whether or not I get sick" may also be as telling as the HLOC.

MBTI

The MBTI provides useful information about underlying issues in the typical dialysis staff member. Both the advantages and pitfalls of their cognitive style are described. A dialysis unit staff that values personal relationships, routine procedures, and caring for those who need them seems ideal.

There are places, however, where the ISFJ personality may find difficulty. Any change in policy or procedure is likely to cause this person hidden distress. The reduction of government funds per person on the units and resulting changes in procedures are likely to be taken as personal affronts by ISFJs. A promotion to head nurse or administration may be experienced as stressful. Because of their desire to maintain traditional values and an emphasis on carrying out standard medical procedures, ISFJ staff members are attractive to a medical unit. Addressing unconscious or countertransference factors in patient care will help the staff avoid any pitfalls in their relationship with patients (Stein 1985).

ISFJs and Death Anxiety

The unexpected death of a patient is likely to be experienced as stressful by the ISFJ. This distress is likely to be dealt with through resignation. ISFJs have a working fatalism for "what happens in life," promoting a tight-knit, traditional view of life and death to others. They are often privately fascinated by more magical or mystical determinants of their future. This dichotomy may be attributed to the ISFJ's orientation to providing care through working with established systems vs. being an advocate of individual needs. They readily give up their concerns to traditions or powers seen to be greater than themselves.

The ISFJ expects patients to follow procedures. The noncompliant patient may be dealt with in the same pattern as the ISFJ's irresponsible spouse. The staff-patient interaction described by "long-suffering, unappreciated staff care" vs. "patient irresponsibility" may perpetuate the noncompliance of the patient. A patient refusing care challenges the ISFJ staff's worldview while eliciting their fascination for someone who does not conform. Any staff disappointments with the unit administration or the ISFJ's worldview may be the source of unwitting behaviors that actually encourage a patient's irresponsibility in treatment.

The ISFJ personality type is not likely to express any overt death anxiety. Face-valid scales such as the Templer Death Anxiety Scale (and the HLC) are not powerful enough to tap the sophisticated defenses of the ISFJ. The most telling symptom of ISFJs' anxiety is their preoccupation with those that seem to flirt with death. Continued patterns of caring or rescuing for persons who are dying is a more sophisticated way to deal with anxiety about death than an attempt to face death directly. This is especially true for ISFJ personalities who hold traditional views that may define life and death in ways that are less broad than their experience.

RECOMMENDATIONS

The higher score on extroverted responses by the registered nurses compared to the technicians suggests the influence of education. Personal awareness and education will prevent destructive staff-patient interactions. Interventions encouraging open communication between staff, patients, and administration are recommended. Assertiveness training inservice workshops, meetings to process thoughts and emotions about any changes on the unit, staffing time devoted to vent emotions and brainstorm about patient care are means to short-circuit any unhealthy messages given to patients by staff. Special attention given to staff impressions regarding a patient's death will encourage staff to be clear and direct with patients and their families about both treatment and death-related issues.

Further research is suggested to demonstrate the cost of the dialysis staff's tendency to internal emotional conflicts. This may be done by measuring patient, staff or administration behavior and attitudes before, during, and after a battery of interventions described above. Research is suggested pairing personality type and health-related behaviors in order to make interventions on a level that is clear and nonthreatening.

REFERENCES

Bradway, K. 1964. "Jung's Psychological Types." *Journal of Analytical Psychology* 9:129-135.

Holmes, C. B. and D. J. Anderson. 1980. "Comparison of Four Death Anxiety Measures." *Psychological Reports* 46:1341-1342.

Jung, C. 1923. *Psychological Types*. New York: Harcourt Brace.

Keirsey, D. and M. Bates. 1984. *Please Understand Me*. Gnosology Books, Ltd.

Lattanner, B. and B. Hayslip. 1984-85. "Occupation-Related Differences in Levels of Death Anxiety." *Omega* 15:53-66.

McCarron, M. L. 1973. "Panel Presentations: Nursing." In A. H. Kutscher and M. R. Goldberg, eds. *Caring for the Dying Patient and His Family*. New York: Health Sciences Publishing Corp.

Myers, I. 1962. *Manual: The Myers-Briggs Type Indicator*. Palo Alto, CA: Consulting Psychologist Press.

Myers, I. 1977. *Supplementary Manual: The Myers-Briggs Type Indicator*. Palo Alto, CA: Consulting Psychologist Press.

O'Dowd, W. 1984-85. "Locus of Control and Level of Conflict as Correlates of Immortality Orientation." *Omega* 15:25-35.

Pettigrew, C. G. and J. G. Dawson. 1979. "Death Anxiety: State or Trait?" *Journal of Clinical Psychology* 35:154-158.

Rotter, J. B. 1966. "Generalized Expectancies for Internal Versus External Control of Reinforcement." *Psychological Monographs* 80 (1, Whole No. 609).

Stein, H. F. 1979. "Rehabilitation and Chronic Illness in American Culture: The Cultural Psychodynamics of a Medical and Social Problem." *Journal of Psychological Anthropology* 2(2):153-176.

Stein, H. F. 1985. *The Psychodynamics of Medical Practice: Unconscious Factors in Patient Care*. Berkeley, CA: University of California Press.

Templer, D. I. 1970. "The Construction and Validation of a Death Anxiety Scale." *The Journal of General Psychology* 82:165-177.

Tolor, A. 1978. "Some Antecedents of Personality Correlates of Health Locus of Control." *Psychological Reports* 43:1159-1165.

Wallston, B. S., K. A. Wallston, G. D. Kaplan, and S. A. Maides. 1976. "Development and Validation of the Health Locus of Control Scale." *Journal of Consulting and Clinical Psychology* 44:580-585.

Willis, C. G. 1982. *Myers-Briggs Type Indicator Tests*. New York: Macmillan.

Implications
for Clinical Anthropology:
Skills for Nurses to Use in Dealing
with Terminal End-Stage Renal Disease
(ESRD) Patients

Jean A. S. MacMullen

Medical anthropology focuses on the cultural dimensions of human life as well as on the biological aspects. The clinically-based medical anthropologist must view a healthy or ill individual in a social situation. Medical anthropologists are assisting health care workers to see their patients as members of complicated networks — social milieus and cultural scenes.

In dealing with renal patients, health care professionals participate in ongoing confrontations with death. As patients go through the myriad of crises confronting them, renal staffs find themselves facing the same questions day in and day out. Staff members may not deal with the problems in so highly personal a manner as their patients do, but due to the constant repetition of patient-related crises, they go through comparable anguish. The more ill a patient becomes, the more staff members must understand his or her support system so as to lessen the patient's alienation and isolation and fulfill their professional responsibilities. The support rendered health care workers by clinical anthropologists has enabled them to view disease not only in a physiological sense but in the psychological, functional, and behavioral sense.

Jean A. S. MacMullen, RN, MS, MA, was former Chief Editor, *Journal of the American Association of Nephrology Nurses and Technicians*, and is currently Assistant Chief, Nursing Service, Veterans Administration Medical Center, Gainesville, FL.

Selective observation and interpretation are the major components of the anthropologist's trade (see Figure 1). Through the incorporation of ethnographic tools, renal staffs have systematically gathered information to guide their patients, their patients' families, and themselves through the stages of terminal illness. Staffs are seeing their patients as individuals through the incorporation of field work. Field work away from the dialysis unit is becoming more popular, but has not become the rule. All renal patients must have holistic workups throughout the phases of their treatment: predialysis workup, treatments as a chronic incenter or home-based patient, terminal illness. Their home physical space, regardless of whether they are a home-based or incenter patient, must be known to all. Their daily life cycle must be recorded and known to all. And last, their biocultural background must be known.

The social network, one of the major components of an ethnography, consists of "patterns of activities and interactions . . . with pathways into the heart of a social system" of an individual (Honigmann 1973, p. 719). Knowledge of the terminally ill patients' social network enables staff members to focus on the kinships, friendships, and patron-client relationships that occur on a day-to-day basis for the patient.

The network shown in Figure 2 represents only one terminally ill

FIGURE 1. Selective Observation and Interpretation (Spradley 1972, p. 14)

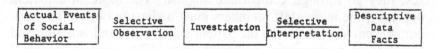

FIGURE 2. Total Network: Paradigmatic Representation

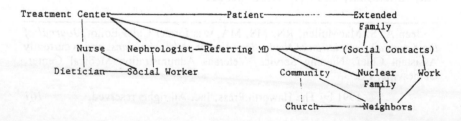

renal patient's social interactions. It demonstrates to the dialysis center's staff how the patient viewed health workers' interaction with him and each other. It also depicts (from the patient's viewpoint) the social contacts within the community and the extended family circle. This network is specific to this patient; each terminally ill patient has his or her own distinctive network. Each patient will view the staff's interactions differently. This patient saw the staff members on an equal plane within his network. This patient and his family shared their fears fully with the staff and were able to deal with death. They worked collaboratively through the patient's initial desire to no longer receive treatments, through the painful weeks of minimal supportive care culminating in a peaceful, dignified death of the patient at home with his family.

Not all networks are as ideal as that shown in Figure 2. The network shown in Figure 3 represents a terminally ill patient who, through personal, cultural, and family stresses, could not cope with the terminal stage of his illness.

Networks like the one depicted in Figure 3 are difficult to record owing to the nonsharing of bonds and lack of cooperation of staff members with each other and with the patient and his family. This network depicts a 60+ year old male with strained family ties (over 30 years of alcohol abuse), no community ties, distrust of medical facilities, and a family whose sole desire was to keep the patient alive so as to maintain their sole source of income. Members of the medical staff were divided by their interpretations of the patient's and his family's desires. The patient became more noncompliant as his condition deteriorated. His family became more angry with the staff because staff members dared to talk about the patient's expressed desires to "die in peace." This patient was maintained on

FIGURE 3. Paradigmatic Representation: Noncoping Patient

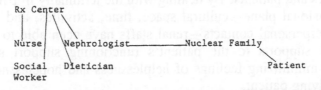

dialysis until his death, by heart failure, following a treatment. The patient's expressed desire to "die in peace" and "not be dialyzed" could not be granted. The patient had been judged mentally incompetent, and his wife named as his legal guardian, more than five years prior to the onset of his renal disease.

The failure of the latter patient to cope with his terminal illness may have been the result of the renal nurses not having the support of a knowledgeable medical anthropologist. The depicted network was developed after the patient's death as a result of an anthropologist's interest in a passing remark made by a nurse. The staff was faced with weak nursing leadership, a sudden inundation of acute patients requiring staff attention and legal restrictions — being judged mentally incompetent, the patient could not take himself off dialysis despite documentation of rational behavior and ability to express his desire for terminating his treatment regimen. One can only speculate that if the latter staff had had the support of the clinically-based anthropologist that the former patient's staff had, staff members would have been able to counsel his family so as to meet his wish for treatment termination.

Since the death of the patient depicted in Figure 3, the nursing staff has gained a permanent head nurse who has incorporated more in-depth data pertaining to social ties, cultural background, and family coping strategies into the unit's patient data base. Furthermore, health workers on the unit have improved lines of communication, which enables them to deal with sudden fluctuations in patient care loads.

Networks like those illustrated are easily recorded. It requires instruction, background reading, and practice. However, the effort expended to gain the expertise can result in cultural sharing and the removal of misunderstandings and conflicts between the health care providers and patients. By dealing with the terminally ill patient on a dimensional plane — cultural space, time, activities, and significant interpersonal contacts — renal staffs have been able to supply external supports to the patient's functioning support system, thereby minimizing feelings of helplessness and hopelessness felt by the dying patient.

REFERENCES

Honigmann, J. J. 1973. *Handbook of Social and Cultural Anthropology*. Chicago: Rand McNally.
Spradley, J. P. 1972. *Culture and Cognition*. New York: Chandler.

ADDITIONAL READING

Mayer, A. C. 1962. *System and Network*. Bombay: Asia Publishing House.
Wolfe, A. W. O. 1970. "On Structural Comparisons of Networks." *Canadian Review of Sociology and Anthropology* 4(7):226-244.

Patient Perceptions
of the Hemodialysis Regimen

H. Katherine O'Neill
Russell E. Glasgow

The medical regimen for patients undergoing chronic hemodialysis is both complex and restrictive. It is therefore not surprising that dialysis patients are not very adherent, particularly to dietary aspects of the regimen. Objective indices of compliance, such as blood chemistry and weight, reveal that only 23-39 percent of dialysis patients consistently follow their dietary recommendations (De-Nour and Czaczkes 1972, 1976; Procci 1978). It has been stated that the major dietary problem is compliance with fluid restrictions (De-Nour and Czaczkes 1976). Nonadherence to this aspect of the regimen is believed to lead to detrimental immediate and long-term effects. During dialysis the "overhydrated" patient is subjected to ultrafiltration, which can result in such physical symptoms as muscle cramps, headache, nausea, and vomiting (Czaczkes and De-Nour 1978; Tyler 1967). Pulmonary edema may also result from excessive overdrinking (Davis, Comty, and Shapiro 1979). Long term effects of excessive fluid intake include more rapid deterioration of cardiac status and greater likelihood of congestive heart failure (Czaczkes and De-Nour 1978). In fact, mortality rates are higher among those renal patients who chronically abuse dietary restrictions than among compliant patients (Abrams, Moore, and Westervelt 1971; De-Nour and Czaczkes 1972).

Considering the numerous ill effects of noncompliance, it is not surprising that treatment programs to increase adherence have be-

H. Katherine O'Neill, MS, is Assistant Professor, Department of Psychology, North Dakota State University, Fargo, ND. Russell E. Glasgow, PhD, is affiliated with the Oregon Research Institute, Eugenia, OR.

gun to appear (Cummings, Becker, and Kirscht 1981; Hart 1979; Magrab and Papadopoulou 1977). It would be helpful in designing interventions to know what difficulties patients encounter in attempting to comply with fluid restrictions, and what strategies they use on their own. Such an approach has proven useful in other problem areas (Perri and Richards 1977) but has not been employed with dialysis patients. Treatment planners might meet with better success if they were aware of patients' perceptions of the regimen and its difficulties before choosing techniques to improve compliance.

It was the intent of this study to investigate patients' views of the hemodialysis regimen, particularly fluid restrictions. We wished to identify the types of barriers that interfere with patients' self-control of fluid intake and to learn what strategies they employ to overcome these barriers.

METHOD

Subjects

Subjects were 26 hemodialysis patients and 13 members of the renal unit nursing staff in a midwestern hospital. All patients were on maintenance dialysis and had been receiving regular treatments for an average of three years (range of one month to nine years). There were 18 men and eight women, with an average age of 53 years (range of 22 to 80 years). Of the sample, 65 percent were married, 23 percent worked either part or full time, and 33 percent reported themselves eligible for kidney transplants. Almost all of the patients (88 percent) reported having received formal instruction in the requirements of the hemodialysis regimen.

There were 31 chronic dialysis patients on the unit at the time the survey was begun. Of these, five were not included in the study: two agreed to participate but underwent kidney transplants before interviews were held; one was deaf and legally blind, so was excluded; and two declined to participate because of poor health.

The 13 staff members who participated in the study included five RNs, five LPNs, a dietician, and two technicians. With the exception of one technician, all were female. The staff members had been working on the renal unit an average of 2.5 years (range of one month to 13 years) and reported direct contact with patients averaging 25 hours per week (range of one to 40 hours weekly). At the time of the study there were 15 members of the hemodialysis nursing staff; two failed to participate for unknown reasons.

Procedure

Two weeks prior to the beginning of the study, all patients were sent a personalized letter describing the project and inviting them to participate. Patients were then approached individually to schedule interviews. Before the interview began, subjects signed an informed consent form stating that the purpose of the project was to "investigate how kidney patients deal with hemodialysis and with restricted lifestyles" and ensuring that all information collected would be kept confidential. The survey was conducted in a combined oral/written format and generally lasted 30 to 45 minutes. (Due to space limitations, only a selected subset of the information collected will be reported in this paper.)

Data collection proceeded differently for renal unit staff members. The project was described by the experimenter at a staff meeting, after which the unit coordinator distributed packets containing consent forms and questionnaires. The nurses were instructed to complete the survey on their own and to avoid discussing it with patients or other staff members.

Measures

The survey items reported herein address three major questions: (1) How difficult and important are fluid restrictions perceived to be? (2) What environmental barriers interfere with fluid control? and (3) What self-control strategies do patients use to achieve adherence?

Three items were used to assess perceptions of the importance and difficulty of restricting fluid intake. First, subjects ranked four general aspects of dialysis according to how problematic they were for patients: feeling thirsty, spending much time on dialysis, physical condition while undergoing dialysis, and physical condition between dialysis sessions. Both patients and staff members ranked these aspects from 1 to 4, with higher values indicating greater difficulty. A second question asked subjects to indicate the relative difficulty of the following dialysis regimen requirements: restricting fluids, restricting sodium, controlling other substances in the diet (e.g., potassium), taking medications, restricting physical activity, and caring for one's cannula or fistula. These items were ranked from "least difficult" to "most difficult" using values from 1 to 6. Finally, subjects rated these same regimen components on their relative importance. Thus, measures were obtained of the perceived difficulty and importance of restricting fluid intake in comparison with other aspects of the dialysis regimen.

Although there has been speculation by health professionals (Comty 1968; Spinozzi 1979), currently there is a scarcity of information from *patients* identifying the types of situations that interfere with compliance to fluid restrictions. Thus, in the present study patients were asked to describe the conditions under which fluid control was most difficult for them. These responses were then categorized into seven major types of situations. Categorizations were made independently by the two authors and agreement was reached in 88 percent of the cases. (When discrepancies occurred, the judgment of the primary author was used.)

In addition to identifying barriers to adherence, patients described the strategies they used in attempting to control fluid intake. These responses were then categorized into eight basic types of strategies. Again, classification was made independently by two raters and 89 percent agreement was reached. (As before, categorizations used by the first author were used when discrepancies occurred.)

Finally, patients' hospital records were examined to determine the number of pounds gained between dialysis sessions. For 17 patients, the average daily weight gain over the previous month was calculated. (Access to the remaining patients' records was not available.) This measure was used as an indirect indicator of compliance with fluid restrictions; greater weight gain would be associated with greater fluid intake and thus with less adherence to recommended guidelines (for this population, approximately 500 ml of fluids daily).

RESULTS

Relative Difficulty and Importance of Fluid Restrictions

In their rank orderings of thirst, time spent in treatment, and physical condition during dialysis and between sessions, patients chose thirst as the most difficult aspect of undergoing chronic dialysis (mean ranking of 3.0 on a 4-point scale). In contrast, staff members rated thirst as the *least* problematic aspect of hemodialysis (mean ranking of 1.9). This represents a statistically significant difference according to a Mann-Whitney U test, $U = 234.5$, $p < .05$. There were no other reliable differences in rankings between patients and nurses.

In rank ordering the requirements of the hemodialysis regimen, patients chose restricting fluid intake as the most difficult (mean ranking of 5.3 on a 6-point scale). Also, patients selected fluid control as the most *important* regimen requirement, although taking medications was a close second (mean rankings of 4.84 and 4.83, respectively). Kidney unit staff members agreed with patients that fluid restrictions were the most important and also the most difficult regimen component.

Barriers to Fluid Control

Patients reported which situations interfered most with their adherence to fluid restrictions and these responses were classified into seven major types. Table 1 lists these categories and the percent of subjects who reported each type of situation as problematic. (Percentages are based on 23 subjects, as three patients did not respond to this item.)

Situations in which food or beverages were being consumed, either by the patient or others, were reported most frequently. These included eating at home or in restaurants, entertaining guests, and attending parties. The second most commonly reported problem was weather conditions. Patients stated that fluid control was most difficult when temperatures were high and/or humidity was low. Other barriers to fluid compliance were time-related. For example, some patients reported feeling thirstier in the mornings or evenings,

TABLE 1. Situations Interfering with Fluid Control

Type of situation	Percent of subjects reporting situation[a]
Food/fluid consumption	56%
Weather	43%
Time-related	26%
Activity level	17%
Dialysis-related	13%
Mood	9%
Miscellaneous	13%

---

[a]Percentages total more than 100% since subjects were free to list as many different situations as they wished

while others experienced greater difficulty with fluid control on weekends as opposed to weekdays. The other problematic situations were related to activity level (e.g., when the subject was either extremely active or inactive), the dialysis process itself (e.g., after a "dry" run), and mood (e.g., when depressed). A final miscellaneous category consisted of specific activities subjects were engaged in (e.g., watching television, smoking) that caused difficulty in controlling fluid intake.

Self-Control Strategies Used

Patients reported using a variety of strategies to control their fluid intake. These techniques were subsequently classified into eight separate types. Table 2 presents these categories and the percent of patients who reported using each type of strategy. (One subject declined to respond to this item, so percentages are based on the remaining 25 subjects.)

TABLE 2. Strategies Used to Control Fluid Intake and Their Correlation with Weight Gain

---

Type of strategy	Percent of subjects using strategy[a]	Correlation with weight gain
Fluid consumption	60%	.18
Pre-planning	40%	.41*
Substitution	32%	-.04
Dietary modification	24%	.22
Situational control	24%	-.28
Distraction	16%	-.47*
Record keeping[b]	8%	---
Miscellaneous	16%	.12

---

[a]Percentages total more than 100% since subjects were free to report as many different strategies as they wished

[b]No correlation computed because weight gain data were unavailable for the subjects using this strategy

*Marginally significant relationship (p < .10)

Interestingly, the first of these, fluid consumption, was the most commonly reported method of self-control. Many patients reported that they dealt with thirst by consuming small amounts of ice or fruit juice. Presumably this strategy prevented them from consuming larger amounts of other liquids. Another popular strategy was preplanning. Examples of this method were premeasuring each day's allowance of liquid or having only certain types of beverages available (e.g., water, soft drinks). Substitution, such as eating fruit or chewing gum, was the third most frequent strategy mentioned. Dietary modification was also used. This usually consisted of avoiding sweet and/or salty foods. Situational control, meaning the avoidance of specific situations that typically led to overdrinking, was also practiced. A few subjects reported distracting themselves or attempting to ignore their thirst. Daily record keeping of fluid intake and weight gain was also described, but by fewer than 10 percent of the sample. Finally, there were some miscellaneous techniques, such as going to bed early to prevent drinking and thinking about the possible detrimental effects of overhydration when tempted to drink.

To determine the general effectiveness of these self-control strategies in preventing fluid overload, point biserial correlations were computed between each type of strategy and weight gain. As shown in Table 2, preplanning methods were apparently unsuccessful; statistical analysis revealed a positive relationship between the use of this strategy and the number of pounds gained. On the other hand, distracting oneself and ignoring thirst was associated with less weight gain between dialysis sessions and appears to be the most successful strategy reported. However, conclusions drawn from these data are limited by the small sample size (N = 16).

DISCUSSION

This study showed that both patients and medical personnel consider fluid restrictions to be one of the most important aspects of the hemodialysis regimen. However, patients perceive thirst as a significant problem and fluid control is thus difficult to achieve. Patients do not appear to be in need of information regarding the importance of following fluid intake recommendations, but do seem to require powerful strategies of self-control.

A number of situations were identified by patients as posing significant barriers to fluid compliance. These cover a wide range of environmental conditions and presumably require a large repertoire of effective self-control techniques. It appears that dialysis patients do employ a variety of self-control strategies, but the effectiveness of these has not been established. Preliminary analysis based on our small sample suggests that some methods may be more helpful than others (e.g., distraction is most strongly associated with smaller weight gains). Similarly, researchers in other areas (i.e., smoking, obesity) have found that certain techniques are more useful in facilitating self-control (Perri and Richards 1977). Among the most effective methods are record keeping, which was only reported by 8 percent of the patients in this survey, and self-reward, which was not reported at all. Interestingly, the most commonly used strategy for fluid control among dialysis patients was actual fluid consumption. That is, patients tended to consume ice or some other liquid in an effort to quench their thirst without excessive fluid intake. It is significant that this method was viewed as a coping response rather than a violation of fluid restrictions. It remains to be investigated whether this strategy actually serves to reduce fluid intake or whether it merely allows patients to rationalize their noncompliance. It also remains to be seen whether patients can be taught to employ different coping skills that will enable them to better overcome the numerous barriers to adherence.

It can be concluded on the basis of this survey that patients, as well as health care professionals, see fluid restrictions as a particularly difficult aspect of the hemodialysis regimen. Furthermore, we have identified a variety of situations that interfere with fluid control. The most common type of situational barrier to compliance — food or beverage consumption in the patient's presence — was reported by over half of the sample. It is likely that similar situations are problematic for dialysis patients elsewhere. Those who design interventions to increase fluid adherence are encouraged to take these data into consideration or, better yet, to collect the same type of information from their own patients. Thus, treatment may be individually tailored to address the particular problems that patients are experiencing.

It may also behoove the initiators of treatment programs to consider which self-control strategies patients are already using to restrict their fluid intake before suggesting coping techniques. While the present study provided initial information on this subject, it failed to provide conclusive evidence for the relative effectiveness of various strategies. Further investigation is warranted before specific self-management techniques are routinely recommended to dialysis patients. As our data suggest, certain methods may be superior and others even detrimental to fluid control. We consider such information to be of great potential value for dialysis patients struggling to adhere to their regimens, as well as for the health professional who is responsible for their care.

REFERENCES

Abrams, H. S., G. L. Moore, and F. B. Westervelt. 1971. "Suicidal Behavior in Chronic Dialysis Patients." *American Journal of Psychiatry* 127:1199-1204.

Comty, C. M. 1968. "Long-Term Dietary Management of Dialysis Patients." *Journal of the American Dieticians Association* 53:439-449.

Cummings K. M., M. H. Becker, and J. P. Kirscht. "Intervention Strategies to Improve Compliance with Medical Regimens by Ambulatory Hemodialysis Patients." *Journal of Behavioral Medicine* 4:111-127.

Czaczkes, J. W. and A. K. De-Nour. 1978. *Chronic Hemodialysis as a Way of Life.* New York: Brunner/Mazel.

Davis, M., C. Comty, and F. Shapiro. 1979. "Dietary Management of Patients with Diabetes Treated by Hemodialysis." *Journal of the American Dietitians Association* 75:265-269.

De-Nour, A. K., and J. W. Czaczkes. 1972. "Personality Factors in Chronic Hemodialysis Patients Causing Noncompliance with Medical Regimen." *Psychosomatic Medicine* 34:333-344.

De-Nour, A. K., and J. W. Czaczkes. 1976. "The Influence of Patients' Personality on Adjustment to Chronic Dialysis." *Journal of Nervous and Mental Disorders* 162:323-332.

Hart, R. R. 1979. "Utilization of Token Economy Within a Chronic Dialysis Unit." *Journal of Consulting and Clinical Psychology* 47:646-648.

Magrab, P. R. and Z. L. Papadopoulou. 1977. "The Effect of a Token Economy on Dietary Compliance for Children on Hemodialysis." *Journal of Applied Behavioral Analysis* 10:575-578.

Perri, M. G. and C. S. Richards. 1977. "An Investigation of Naturally Occurring Episodes of Self-Controlled Behaviors." *Journal of Counseling Psychology* 24:178-183.

Procci, W. R. 1978. "Dietary Abuse in Maintenance Hemodialysis Patients." *Psychosomatics* 19:16-24.

Spinozzi, N. S. 1979. "Teaching Nutritional Management to Children on Hemodialysis." *Journal of the American Dieticians Association* 75:157-159.

Tyler, H. R. "Neurological Complications in Uremia." In A. R. Brest and J. H. Moyer, eds. *Renal Failure.* Philadelphia, J. B. Lippincott Co.

V. RENAL DISEASE
AND SPECIAL PATIENT POPULATIONS

AIDS and End-Stage Renal Disease: Issues of Our Times

Robert S. Lampke

As the number of cases of AIDS (acquired immune deficiency syndrome) increases and as more is known about various manifestations of the illness, cases are being reported of AIDS patients who develop renal failure and go on to require hemodialysis. At the same time cases are also being reported of patients with end-stage renal disease (ESRD) who either develop AIDS or are found to be antibody positive — that is, to have been exposed to the AIDS virus.

AIDS OVERVIEW

Acquired immune deficiency syndrome (AIDS) has been referred to by some as the number one health problem in the United States

Robert S. Lampke, MD, is Clinical Assistant Professor of Psychiatry, SUNY Health Sciences Center at Brooklyn, and is Attending Psychiatrist, Consultation-Liaison Service, State University Hospital, Brooklyn, NY.

The author thanks the medical and nursing staff of the Hemodialysis Service and of the Renal Transplant Service at Kings County Hospital Center — State University Hospital for their observations, comments and assistance in the preparation of this manuscript. Special thanks are extended to Dr. T.K.S. Rao, Ms. Sutton, Ms. B. Siegel, Ms. McCall, and Dr. M. DelMonte.

today. It is a major life-threatening illness, strikes relatively healthy and young patients in the prime of their lives, has no known cure, and carries a very high mortality rate within two to three years of diagnosis.

AIDS is an infectious disease characterized by the presence of opportunistic infections in someone with no known cause of an immune compromised state and an inverted T4/T8 ratio.

Aids related complex (ARC) is the presence of some of the characteristics of the illness but with no opportunistic infections.

Human immunodeficiency virus (HIV) is the etiologic agent responsible for AIDS; it is lymphotrophic as well as neurotrophic, meaning that it attacks lymphocytes and nervous tissue cells.

ELISA — enzyme-linked immunosorbent assay — tests the presence of antibodies to the HIV virus. It does not tell if one has or will develop AIDS. *The Western Blot test* is a more specific and more expensive test.

Transmission of the virus is mainly by sexual intercourse with an infected person, by infected blood or blood products, or from an infected mother to the fetus or newborn. It is spread by direct blood-to-blood or semen-to-blood contact.

Groups at risk for AIDS include homosexual or bisexual men, intravenous drug abusers (both past and present), and sex partners of the above. According to the latest estimates, these groups account for 95 percent of all cases in the United States (U.S. Public Health Service and WHO 1987).

There have been over 35,000 reported cases of AIDS in the United States and more than 20,000 deaths; about 100,000 people are estimated to have ARC and 1.5 million people to be infected with the AIDS virus (HIV antibody positive). Seven percent of patients with ARC go on to develop AIDS yearly and about 20 to 30 percent of those who are HIV positive develop AIDS within five years or about 10 percent per year (Sullivan 1987; Bobbey 1987).

ESRD OVERVIEW

End-stage renal disease (ESRD) or complete loss of kidney function is most commonly caused by chronic kidney disease. Advances in medical technology have now made it possible to maintain patients on artificial kidney machines. This procedure is referred to as hemodialysis (HD) or peritoneal dialysis (PD). Another treatment is a kidney transplant, referred to as renal transplantation.

It is estimated that there are currently about 75,000 patients on dialysis and that about 5,000 renal transplants are done each year in the United States alone (Cummings and Klahr 1985).

Renal Manifestations in AIDS

Kidney failure in AIDS patients can be divided into three groups: Group 1, acute renal failure; Group 2, immune complex, glomerulonephritis; and Group 3, chronic renal failure (AIDS-associated nephropathy).

Acute renal failure is potentially reversible and is due to (a) acute tubular necrosis from prolonged renal ischemia secondary to such etiologies as hypotension, hypovolemia, respiratory failure, radiologic contrast agents and nephrotoxic antibiotics; and (b) allergic interstitial nephritis from drugs and other antibiotics. Immune complex glomerulonephritis is possibly related to septic complications of AIDS.

AIDS-associated nephropathy is a form of chronic renal failure characterized by massive proteinuria, focal and segmental glomerulosclerosis (FSGS) and rapid deterioration in renal function to end-stage uremia in 8-16 weeks. The lesion is similar to that of heroin-associated nephropathy previously reported by Rao and associates (1984) where onset to uremia occurred within 7-72 months and the mean duration to onset was 7.1 months. Idiopathic FSGS goes to renal failure in two to three years.

Patients with ESRD may be exposed to the AIDS virus by membership in a high-risk group, e.g., homosexuals/bisexuals or intravenous drug abusers, or through transfusion or organ transplant.

In one large series of patients with AIDS, 78 of 750 AIDS patients (10.4 percent) were evaluated for renal problems. Reversible acute renal failure — Group I — was found in 23 (30 percent). AIDS-associated nephropathy was found in the remaining 55 (70 percent), and irreversible uremia developed in 43. There were an additional 18 patients with a history of intravenous drug abuse in whom AIDS was diagnosed subsequent to starting maintenance hemodialysis.

Only two of the patients with AIDS-associated nephropathy survived more than two months. All of the ESRD patients who developed AIDS died within three months of the diagnosis of AIDS. Death followed a syndrome of failure to thrive in the patients with AIDS-associated nephropathy and in the ESRD patients who developed AIDS.

The authors conclude that maintenance hemodialysis is not efficacious in significantly prolonging life in either patients with AIDS-associated nephropathy and uremia or in patients with ESRD who develop AIDS during the course of maintenance hemodialysis. AIDS patients who have potentially irreversible acute renal failure may, however, benefit from hemodialysis (Rao et al. 1987).

There have been several reports of HIV testing done on groups of both dialysis and renal transplant patients (Goldman et al. 1986; Margreiter et al. 1986; Neumayer, Wagner, and Kresse 1986). One hundred patients on hemodialysis were tested for the AIDS antibody. Eight had positive ELISA and five had a positive Western Blot. Two of these were in high-risk groups and the other three had a history of multiple transfusions. Another study tested 115 cadaveric recipients, ten of whom had a positive or questionable ELISA; only one was confirmed as positive. The kidney donor had a history of intravenous drug abuse and the recipient of the other kidney tested positive also. Other cases of HIV positivity in renal transplant recipients were traced to blood transfusions and to the transplanted kidney. The impression from reviewing these articles is that the risk of AIDS in HD patients is low. As of now there is no data on how asymptomatic HIV positive patients on hemodialysis do.

There also have been some interesting observations concerning AIDS and hemodialysis (Klein 1986). Among them is the observation that renal failure impairs host defenses, including cell-mediated immunity, and that the Center for Disease Control (CDC) definition of AIDS includes the absence of other causes of immunodeficiency. This would preclude the diagnosis of AIDS in patients with renal failure; however, with the antibody test, the diagnosis of AIDS can better be made.

Another observation is that immunosuppressive therapy reduces, and rejection episodes enhance, virus propagation. It may be that cyclosporin reduces replication of HIV. It has been suggested to avoid measures that stimulate immune response and, in HIV-positive transplant recipients, not to withdraw immunosuppressive therapy (Margreiter et al. 1986).

COPING WITH ESRD

The way a patient copes with an illness depends on three major factors—biological, psychological, and social. Biological aspects include symptoms, course, and complications, especially of the Central Nervous System (CNS). Psychological aspects include previous level of psychological adjustment and personality integration. Social refers to social supports as well as sociocultural stigma attached to the illness and afflicted groups (Wellisch 1985).

Coping ability depends on how many areas are affected; if one area is affected, coping is potentially reduced; if two areas, moderately; if all three areas are affected, coping is severely reduced (Levy 1979a).

Before examining how patients with ESRD cope with AIDS and how patients with AIDS cope with ESRD, it will be helpful to review briefly what we know in general about coping with the two illnesses.

End-stage renal disease, as the name says, is the end stage of chronic renal disease; those affected have had a significant length of time to adjust to the course of the illness, its prognosis and treatment.

Biological factors. ESRD is the last stage of a chronic illness, and patients generally have been sick and then gotten better or worse with dialysis or renal transplantation. Treatment extends their life expectancy; patients are chronically and severely anemic and intermittently uremic; they are prone to infections and there is a mortality of about 10 percent per year.

ESRD is caused by a variety of diseases. In addition to the progression of the renal disease, patients also experience the symptoms and complications of these underlying diseases and their treatments, such as vascular lesions and peripheral neuropathy from chronic diabetes, or side effects from antihypertensive medications. For the male patient there is the added stress of the loss of urination from the male sex organ, which may decrease his sense of masculinity.

Psychological factors. Psychological factors that facilitate adjustment to dialysis include an ability to regress and to tolerate being dependent on others, in particular the dialysis treatment and the treatment team.

Patients who protest their independence and who cannot tolerate the dependent role may react by being depressed or anxious or by not cooperating in treatment. This is especially so for the adolescent facing the developmental tasks of independence and autonomy.

On the other hand the very dependent patient may "enjoy" his dependence and be reluctant to give it up and to fully cooperate in rehabilitation and become more independent outside of the dialysis treatments. This has implications for treatment in that the more independent patient may do better on home dialysis or by having a renal transplant (Levy 1979a; Stewart 1984).

Social factors. Some patients are disabled and not able to work. As a result there are job and family stresses and role reversals. For example, if the man is disabled and not able to work, he commonly stays home and becomes active in household activities while the woman goes to work. This may be seen as a threat to the man's sense of masculinity, especially if it was dependent on his gender role prior to becoming sick (Levy 1979b).

There are, however, self-help support groups on both the local and national level for dialysis patients; in addition there are organizations such as the National Association of Hemodialysis and Renal Transplantation Patients.

Stresses of Chronic Hemodialysis

Patients with ESRD who are on maintenance hemodialysis are literally dependent on the machine. Treatment consists of being hooked up to the machine for treatments of four to six hours in duration, about three times a week. Some patients become anxious at the sight of seeing their blood circulate outside of their body, into the machine and back into their body. Others become fearful that the machine will fail or malfunction. Males have been known to masturbate in an attempt to deal with their high anxiety. There are also dietary and fluid restrictions that place further constraints and stresses on their functioning. Patients use a variety of defense mechanisms to help them cope with dialysis—among them denial, projection, and displacement (De-Nour 1976; Levy 1979a).

Psychological syndromes seen in patients with ESRD include both organic and functional disorders.

Encephalopathy with Renal Disease

Encephalopathies associated with renal disease can either be due to renal disease per se or to a complication of its treatments. They include uremic encephalopathy, dialysis dementia, dialysis disequilibration syndrome, and treatment-related Wernicke-Korsakoff syndrome (Comomy 1982). Uremic encephalopathy is from renal disease per se, the other three are from complications of treatment of chronic renal failure.

Uremic encephalopathy is similar to other organic brain syndromes (OBS) in that there is a fluctuation in course and symptoms. Among the prominent clinical signs are disorientation, slurred speech, mental confusion, and slowed thought processes. The treatment is supportive measures and dialysis or renal transplant. Dialysis brings down the elevated blood urea nitrogen (BUN).

Dialysis dementia is a progressive dementia with psychotic features such as delusions and hallucinations; often there is an associated agitation. In addition there is a dysarthric speech characterized by stuttering and stammering, myoclonus and multifocal and generalized seizures. The cause is unknown; there is speculation that aluminum may play a role. It lasts from one month to three years, with an average of six months before death ensues.

Dialysis disequilibration syndrome is more common with rapid hemodialysis; it is frequent during dialysis but may not show until 24 hours after a run. The cause is believed to be pathological shifts of water into the brain. The treatment is to reduce fluid overload by fluid restriction.

Wernicke-Korsakoff syndrome is a confusional-amnestic syndrome that develops in patients who have not received supplemental thiamine.

Adjustment to Renal Transplantation

Prior to a renal transplant operation, there is often a denial of the severity of illness, and patients seem apathetic. This is contrasted with feeling hopeful at the prospect of receiving a kidney transplant and the opportunity to be liberated from dependence on the dialysis machine. In exchange for this freedom from the machine, patients now have to be on immunosuppressive medications, which carry with them a new set of side effects and potential complications. Other psychological factors include donor motivation, the psychological relationship between the donor and the recipient, and feelings and attitudes toward receiving a cadaver transplant (Dubovsky and Penn 1980; Eisendrath 1976; Steinberg and Levy 1979).

Postoperative psychological factors are comprised of body image changes, which can be functional (emotional) or organic in etiology, for example, facial and/or bodily changes secondary to side effects of immunosuppressive medications. Likewise, depression and psychosis can be organic or functional in nature (Steinberg and Levy 1979).

In discussing the rejection of a transplanted kidney, the possible contributory role of psychological factors such as hopelessness and helplessness should be kept in mind (Steinberg and Levy 1979).

Behavioral problems. This includes the acting out of aggression by becoming angry with the dialysis staff on whom the patient has become dependent by reason of the frequent treatments. Other responses may include missing appointments and treatments, binge eating, and fluid overload. At times there can be suicidal behavior out of a sense of frustration with the chronicity of illness and the need for continual treatments (De-Nour 1976).

Compliance problems. These include noncompliance with medications, dialysis treatments, and dietary and fluid restrictions. Some of the factors contributing to noncompliance have been discussed by Stewart (1984). They include: characterological problems, denial of illness, psychological gain from the sick role, suicidal behavior, dysfunctional family, irrational prejudices, and problems with body image.

A decision to withdraw from hemodialysis can be seen as a final compliance problem; however there may be other causes, for example, a rational decision that the quality of life on dialysis is not satisfactory, a manipulative gesture done out of anger at family members, or a severe depression.

As mentioned previously, there are no data on the prognosis of asymptomatic HIV positive patients on hemodialysis. If they are not members of high risk groups such as homosexuals or drug addicts, and acquired the AIDS virus through blood transfusions or organ transplants, they are likely to be angry and feel that they are innocent victims.

COPING WITH AIDS

As stated previously, the way a patient copes with an illness depends on three areas—medical or biological, psychological, and social. Many AIDS patients are affected in the medical and social areas. There are frequent and debilitating infections, often of the Central Nervous System (CNS). These impair patients' ability to function and often affect their memory and emotions.

These infections of the CNS may be due to direct invasion of the brain by the AIDS virus or by an opportunistic infection, for example, toxoplasmosis. This may cause either confusional states or dementia-like pictures. This has been referred to as AIDS encephalopathy and AIDS dementia. CT scans of the head commonly show dilated ventricles and cerebral atrophy while the EEG shows generalized slowing (Delley, Shelp, and Batki 1986).

There is a great deal of stigma attached not only to the disease but also to the two main groups that are affected by the illness, namely, homosexual men and intravenous drug abusers. Some have said that AIDS victims belong to groups that are in some ways social outcasts—homosexuals, drug addicts, Haitian immigrants. An article in the *Village Voice* ("AIDS and Race" 1987) notes that there is a marked lack of sympathy for drug users among people who have been victims of drug-related crime.

Psychiatric Manifestations of AIDS

The psychiatric manifestations of AIDS, especially some of the early signs of brain damage ("Psychological Sequelae" 1985), include persistent headaches, difficulty concentrating, a "sloweddown feeling," lack of interest, and withdrawal. Looking at the list, one could say that the patient is depressed and one would miss an organic etiology. Here a brain wave tracing-EEG might show slowing that would help to confirm the diagnosis.

Psychiatric syndromes that have been seen in AIDS patients include:

Functional

Anxiety reactions
Depression
Suicidal behaviors

Organic Brain Syndromes

Delirium
Dementia

The organic brain syndromes have been mentioned above. It is helpful to have a high index of suspicion that psychiatric manifestations may be organic in etiology.

As with other terminal illnesses, psychological reactions in patients with AIDS are more frequent and more intense at certain points in the course of the illness. These include but are not limited to the following: HIV antibody testing, time of diagnosis, discharge from hospital, relapse, and terminal phase.

Psychological reactions to HIV testing will be discussed in detail below. Reactions to the diagnosis or suspected diagnosis of AIDS are frequently so strong that there is often a stress response syndrome with alternating intense anxiety and emotional numbing; there may also be suicidal ideation. This crisis stage is followed by transitional stages characterized by such reactions as anger, confusion, and distress (Nichols 1985). It is not uncommon at this stage, when patients need all the support they can get, that family and friends may reject and abandon them out of their fears of contracting the illness.

Depression is one of the more common reasons for requesting psychiatric consultation on AIDS patients, and adjustment disorder with depressed mood was the most frequent psychiatric diagnosis in one series (Delley et al. 1985).

I asked the head nurse and doctors of several dialysis units how patients with AIDS cope with hemodialysis. Their observations follow:

First of all, there was a difference as to where in the hospital dialysis was done with AIDS patients. At one hospital, dialysis treatments were done in a single room, on a general medical floor or even on the medical prison ward. At another hospital, dialysis was done in the corridor outside the regular dialysis unit. A third hospital used the isolation/hepatitis room on the dialysis unit.

Some facilities are just beginning to have experience with AIDS patients who develop renal failure. At one hospital, AIDS patients on dialysis were primarily intravenous drug abusers, with only a few homosexuals. Some patients were hostile and not tolerant of the treatment. For example, some were prisoners who were so hostile over having contracted AIDS that they said they would "give it to the medical and nursing staff" before leaving the prison ward. This calls to mind a *New York Times* report ("Inmates Put Serum in Coffee" 1986) about prisoners putting blood serum from an AIDS patient in a guard's coffee. This behavior is in part due to the premorbid character of these prisoners and in part to anger at having this fatal illness.

Intravenous drug abusers who have developed ESRD and then gotten well with dialysis are not so hostile when they develop AIDS, probably because they have had time to adjust to ESRD. They have already passed through the stages of psychological adaptation to hemodialysis: "honeymoon," disenchantment and discouragement, and long-term adaptation (Levy 1977).

The patient with AIDS is generally quite ill from AIDS when he develops renal failure; he may have a fever, cough, or pneumonia. He wants to feel better but there does not seem to be any honeymoon period. Furthermore, he knows that he is going to die from AIDS as there is no known cure.

According to another hospital, patients with AIDS were no different from other dialysis patients.

A doctor at a third hospital said some of the patients with AIDS who went on to develop renal failure were neurologically impaired and some seemed too confused to fully understand the treatments.

Coping with HIV Testing

As mentioned previously, there are two tests for the presence of antibodies to the AIDS virus. Initial testing is done with the ELISA test. Positive results are confirmed with a second ELISA and/or with the Western Blot, a more expensive and specific test. Ninety percent of positive ELISA done on routine screened healthy adults are found to be negative with Western Blot. So if individuals who are not members of a high-risk group are told of a positive ELISA before it is confirmed with the Western Blot, nine out of ten of them will be alarmed unnecessarily (McKegney 1986).

It should be kept in mind that the ELISA and Western Blot are not tests for AIDS but for presumed exposure to the virus. They were initially developed to screen infected blood and are now used to verify and support a diagnosis of AIDS. As mentioned previously, they do not tell if one has AIDS or if one will develop AIDS. The clinical significance is unclear, but someone who is HIV antibody positive is presumed to be infectious to others. About 20-30 percent of HIV positive individuals go on to develop AIDS in two to five years or at a rate of about 10 percent per year (T.K.S. Rao, personal communication, 1 January 1987).

Benefits. There should be a specific reason to do the test. What does one do with the results? Will a positive result help confirm a suspected diagnosis in a patient critically ill with multiple opportunistic infections? There is no reason to do the test if someone discontinues using drugs and is not pregnant or planning to get married and have a baby. You may want to do the test if a female drug addict wants to have a baby, change her behavior, and/or discontinue a pregnancy. People in high-risk groups should consider themselves to be infected and potentially contagious. In some institutions the doctors can't get the results directly but only with the patient's permission (Bihari et al. 1986).

There is a lot of ambivalence over test results and how the information will be used. For example, will a positive result cause a proposed marriage to be cancelled or an established one to be terminated? With babies of high-risk groups, foster agencies often do not want to do testing as they do not know what they will do with the results (Bihari et al. 1986).

With respect to ESRD, some hemodialysis units may want to do mass testing of their patients. Such an approach ignores the potential for adverse effects to be incurred by the patient.

Risks. There are profound consequences from HIV testing. One major issue has to do with confidentiality—who has access to the results and what will they be used for? For example, is it an infringement on personal freedom for an insurance company to insist on HIV testing as a prerequisite for insuring someone? Another issue is the disruptive effect on a person's life of a positive or even a false positive (until confirmed) test result. This is even more important since the person may never come down with AIDS.

HIV counseling. One hour of precounseling is recommended to advise the person of the risks, benefits, and consequences of HIV testing. As with genetic counseling, the idea is to present information without recommending or coercing the person into taking the test. The testing process should be voluntary, confidential, and non-coercive.

Post-test counseling should also be available to help the person cope with the significance and impact of a positive test result as well as the testing process.

Generally speaking, individuals react with increased anxiety to HIV testing. There are, however, differences as to how gay men and IVDA's respond to the testing process. Table 1 lists some of these differences (Bihari et al. 1986; National Institutes of Mental Health 1986).

Case Examples

The following two case vignettes will illustrate the profound consequences that can occur with HIV testing.

Case 1. A patient with a long history of ESRD had been on HD for the past seven years. He had a history of intravenous drug abuse

Table 1. Psychological Impact of HIV Antibody Testing

Defense Mechanisms and Responses

Gay Men	IVDA
Mature Defenses	Primitive Defenses
Healthy Egos	Damaged Egos
Internal Locus of Control	External Locus of Control
Responses: Adaptation, Peer Groups	Denial, Projection
Reach Out, Sublimate, Altruism	Act Out, Increase Drug Use
At Times increase in Sex Behavior	Psychotic Regression
Generally Limit Sexual Behavior	Suicidal Behavior

and had become increasingly depressed after being told by his dialysis center that he tested positive for the AIDS virus. Even though he had no symptoms of AIDS, he eventually came to believe that he had AIDS. His aunt died and shortly thereafter his mother died. After that he became suicidal, left his hotel, got high on drugs and then tried to kill himself with an overdose of cocaine. He was brought to the hospital, treated on the medical service for the overdose and then transferred to the psychiatric service for treatment of depression. He continued to receive dialysis in the hospital while on both the medical and psychiatric services.

Case 2. Following chest surgery a patient was found to have an unusual bacteria that had only been reported three times in the literature. The infectious disease specialist wanted to test the patient for the AIDS virus. He spent an hour with him telling him that although he had no symptoms of AIDS it would be "to his advantage" to have the test done. Following this discussion the patient became increasingly anxious, then withdrawn, and ended up refusing all food, medication, and treatments. Over the next three days he developed a brief reactive psychosis and had to be transferred to the psychiatric service. There he remained for the next two weeks until the psychosis resolved. Here the test was being done more for the benefit of the doctor than the patient, and even if it were positive, it would not have changed the patient's treatment (Bihari et al. 1986).

These two case vignettes illustrate rather dramatically that HIV testing is not without risk and should be done only for valid clinical reasons.

SOCIAL CLIMATE SURROUNDING AIDS

The social climate surrounding an illness or disease is determined by various factors, among them the disease itself, how serious or devastating it is, how it is spread and by what types of contact. Is it contagious? Is there a cure for it? How is it viewed by the medical community, the media, and the political community?

AIDS is an infectious disease that has no known cure and a very high mortality within two to three years of diagnosis. To the best of current medical knowledge, transmission is by two main routes. The first is by sexual contact with infected males such as occurs with homosexual/bisexual males and their sexual partners. The other route is among drug addicts who share dirty needles and thus transmit the virus in the blood. Less frequent ways are through receiving infected blood products such as occurs among hemophiliacs. This latter route has become much less frequent with improved blood testing and the development of nonhuman blood products.

Impact on Health Care Workers

This has not lessened the fears of the general as well as the medical community about the spread of AIDS, although some of the early hysteria seems to have died down as more is known about the illness and new ways of transmission have not been discovered. A sample of some of the headlines that have appeared in the local media over the last several years includes: "Public's Anxiety and Reality on Blood Transfusion"; "AIDS: Deadly But Hard to Catch"; "A.M.A. Says Students With AIDS Should Not Be Barred by Schools"; "AIDS Hospice Stirs Controversy"; "Patient Gets AIDS Virus Despite Blood Test"; "Co-Workers Walk Off Jobs As an AIDS Victim Returns"; "World Drive on an AIDS 'Pandemic'"; "Nurses Quit Jobs, Won't Treat AIDS Patients"; "Morticians Won't Bury AIDS Victims"; "Surgeons Won't Operate on Victims of AIDS"; "Anti-AIDS Bias by Undertakers Ruled a Human Rights Breach."

All this press cannot help but have some effect on health care workers.

Some of the impact of AIDS on health care workers has to do with the physical and emotional stresses of caring for dying patients. This includes working with patients who are generally young, at an age when one is generally not expected to come down with a fatal and incurable disease. There are also the stresses of dealing with families and lovers.

The added impact that AIDS has on health care workers is the fear of contracting an illness that has no known cure and a high mortality; this may at times affect their ability to care for AIDS patients. They may avoid or minimize time spent with patients.

At one hospital that has been working with AIDS patients since 1982, only one staff member initially volunteered to work with the

AIDS patients on HD as she had no fear of getting AIDS. Some of the other staff did not want to work with them, but the hospital administrator told them they had to take turns working with the AIDS patients. It was also beneficial to have staff from the infectious disease department talk with them about the illness to allay their fears and to reassure them that they can't catch it from casual contact. Until more is known about the transmission, the staff know that they have to be careful with needles and to observe necessary precautions and safeguards. (This will be discussed in greater detail in the section on giving HD to patients with AIDS.)

Similar observations were noted at other HD units including a university outpatient HD unit and a voluntary hospital HD unit.

The head nurse and the assistant head nurse at a university renal transplant unit told me that their staff and patients do not have the same fears and concerns about AIDS that the HD staff do.

Effect on Quality of Patient Care

At one hospital, AIDS patients were dialyzed in a single room on the medical floor using strict sterile and isolation technique. When one patient needed HD, the staff wanted him to move to a single room. He refused as it had no air conditioning and he felt the room was too confining. The hospital staff then literally moved him in his bed to this single room. He responded by walking back to his original room and lying down on another empty bed. He told the staff that the Patient's Bill of Rights said that a patient's bed could not be changed without his or her permission.

At this point a psychiatric consultation was requested to assess his competency to refuse treatment, but the real issue was over whether he could refuse a single room. He was agreeable to being dialyzed in the single room but didn't want to stay there. He later agreed to move into the single room when the staff agreed to repair the air conditioning. Issues relating to the loss of control and autonomy faced by a dying patient came up later in his care. Another AIDS-related issue emerged when he tried to get the light bulbs changed in his room. When told that the electricians could not fix the lights he said, "How can they say that, they never came into my room to try?'' It came out that no electrician wanted to change the light bulbs in the room of an AIDS patient until that patient had been moved out.

Health care workers have not developed AIDS from routine care of AIDS patients. There have been seven separate studies in the United States and Great Britain on the outcome of needle stick injuries and other exposures such as to eyes or nostrils. Out of 1500 health care workers, the five with evidence of the HIV virus in their blood had had severe exposure by deep injection wound or puncture from a grossly contaminated large bore biopsy needle. None with direct exposure of mucous membranes to blood or other body fluids developed HIV infections. To date there is also no evidence that the virus is transmitted by human bites, food, or insects. Nurses who have given mouth-to-mouth resuscitation also showed no evidence of infection (National Institutes of Mental Health 1986).

The most impressive study to date is a study of approximately 105 persons in close personal contact with AIDS patients at home. Of the contacts who did not have sex with the AIDS patients, only one had evidence of infection and that was probably transmitted from the mother to the infant in pregnancy (National Institutes of Mental Health 1986).

Effect on Public Policy/Funding

With a continuing increase in the number of new AIDS cases, continuing care and treatment of existing cases, and the continuing search for a vaccine and for new treatments, the AIDS epidemic has major implications in public policy/funding in the areas of health, budget, and testing.

With particular reference to AIDS and ESRD, hemodialysis is done two to three times per week. At one municipal hospital the costs for HD are included in a single daily rate, whereas at a state university medical center the cost for HD is separate. The issue of who pays for AIDS is a controversial one and is becoming problematic for the insurance industry. Some insurance companies have tried to deny health or life insurance to people who are HIV positive. In 1985 the Center for Disease Control (CDC) projected hospital costs for AIDS patients to average $147,000. A high-risk pool made up of contributions from insurance companies, similar to that for other chronic illnesses such as diabetes and cystic fibrosis has been suggested ("AIDS: Deadly" 1986).

As mentioned previously, a positive antibody test does not mean that the person will get the illness. One health economist has estimated that the total lifetime cost of hospitalization for a patient with AIDS ranged from $60,000 to $75,000 in 1984 or about half the $147,000 cost per patient that was projected last year by the CDC. Put in a larger perspective, this amount is less than half the $158,000 lifetime cost of providing medical care and dialysis to a patient with ESRD. In addition, the AIDS expense will represent .3 percent of the country's total direct health costs of $454.2 billion for 1986 ("Who Pays" 1986). In the early days of dialysis, treatments were done only on patients who had no other illnesses. Now that treatment is more available, it is done on patients if the patient and family so desire, even in the presence of other illnesses. So whether the patient has AIDS or not should not be a deciding factor. As mentioned earlier in this paper, there is a poor prognosis for patients with AIDS who develop AIDS-associated nephropathy as well as for patients with ESRD who go on to develop AIDS. Treatment of such patients should be decided on a case-by-case basis in discussion with the patient and his family (T.K.S. Rao, personal communication, 1 January 1987).

The HD staff at one hospital did have concerns about doing HD on AIDS patients. They felt that since these patients are so ill and emaciated and have such a poor prognosis (in that they generally die within a few months), why should their suffering be prolonged? Does HD really improve the quality of their life? Furthermore, there was concern about the risk of exposing the HD staff to the AIDS virus.

TECHNOLOGY, TRANSFUSIONS AND TRANSPLANTS: THE EFFECT OF AIDS ON PATIENTS WITH ESRD

Before the advances of modern medical technology, patients with ESRD had a shortened life expectancy. Although the disease still cannot be cured, with hemodialysis and renal transplantation patients can enjoy a longer life and are able to be more independent and even to travel.

To the already present risks of contracting hepatitis and other infections in an immunocompromised state, there are now the added risks and fears of contracting AIDS from blood transfusions and organ transplants. What have been some of the responses of patients with ESRD to the AIDS problem?

One response has been that ESRD patients do not want to have blood transfusions until absolutely necessary; they prefer to "wait it out" or to receive blood substitutes. Some have had to have transfusions due to very low hematocrits; then the staff has to reassure the patients that the blood has been tested for the AIDS virus. Some patients needing renal biopsies would not agree to allow themselves to receive a transfusion during the biopsy if it became a medical necessity, and as a result the biopsies were not done.

At one hospital dialysis patients previously accepted the need for transfusions without question; now they question the need and ask what are the chances of getting AIDS. A diabetic renal transplant self-help group asks for reassurance that organ donors are fully tested.

Another hospital dialyzes AIDS patients in isolation rooms on the HD unit; they have observed that this upsets the other patients who see the AIDS patients and the HD staff in masks, gloves, and gowns.

I was unable to obtain any evidence that patients are delaying receiving renal transplants out of fear of receiving an infected kidney. At present there is hope for new technological advances in treatment, such as recombinant erythropoietin, that can reduce the need for blood transfusions ("Cost of AIDS Care" 1986). There is also new research on renal transplantation that shows that transfusions do not significantly impact on the outcome; as a result, one renal transplant unit is backing off on insisting on the need for pre-transplant transfusions.

Patient Education

The key here is to have different medical specialists talk with the patient about their concerns. This may mean an infectious disease specialist or a blood bank director. In one instance a rather sophisticated and highly educated diabetic renal transplant self-help group wanted to know if the immune deficiency state in AIDS was similar to that of immune compromised renal transplant patients. A research immunologist was called in to answer their questions and concerns.

In addition to providing patients with information, they should be continuously reassured and reminded that blood products and organs for transplantation are routinely tested for the HIV virus.

Guidelines for the Renal Community

General precautions. At present it is being recommended that the precautions that have been developed against Hepatitis B be used. This includes blood precautions and techniques for preventing needle-stick injuries and avoiding contact with bodily secretions ("Synthesized Drug" 1986).

HIV Screening. This is not indicated routinely for HD patients and staff. Blood transfusions and organ transplants both from live donors and from cadaveric donors are all being tested for the HIV antibody. Counseling and treatment of HIV positive patients should also be available (Center for Disease Control 1986).

Recommendations for giving hemodialysis to AIDS patients. The dialysis machines should be disinfected and sterilized. It is not necessary to isolate patients if the precautions for Hepatitis B are followed ("Synthesized Drug" 1986), though this may be advisable for the peace of mind of other patients and staff. Sometimes isolation with the attendant gowns, gloves, and masks has an upsetting effect on other patients. If the patient is critically ill and in the hospital, it is probably advisable to administer HD in a separate area or room using isolation techniques.

TREATMENT AND PREVENTION OF AIDS

It is beyond the scope of this paper to address fully the topic of treatment and prevention of AIDS. However, some general comments will be given.

The treatment of AIDS patients involves treatment of opportunistic infections, as there is no known cure. There is hope that a vaccine will be discovered in the future. There is also a lot of hope that

AZT (azothymidine) will be effective in treating infections. Other treatments include nutritional therapies, multidisciplinary teams who also try to find appropriate places for AIDS patients to go after they no longer need to be in the hospital. The post-hospital disposition of AIDS patients continues to be a problem as there are many patients who are no longer wanted by their families.

Prevention is a broad area of discussion and involves many different aspects. Some pertain to technological advances, others to social, moral, and ethical issues. Infection control measures have been mentioned previously. An example of technological advances would be improvements in testing for the presence of the HIV virus in blood and organs and ways of predicting who might come down with the illness. Who should be tested and should there be mandatory testing, for example, of army recruits, health insurance applicants, marriage license applicants, convicted rapists, and prostitutes? Who should have access to the results?

Public health efforts need to be directed to reducing the spread of AIDS. Efforts in the gay community should be directed to bringing about changes in sexual behavior, especially to reduce the excessive number of sexual partners that characterized some of the permissiveness of the late 1970s and early 1980s. Also, "safe sex" should be reinforced — personal hygiene, use of condoms, and preventing or limiting the exchange of bodily and sexual fluids. There is a large advertising effort to advise the general public about measures to prevent the spread of AIDS; this involves such aspects as condom advertising on television and in the newspapers as well as free distribution of condoms in singles bars and theaters. Some television networks have refused to carry condom ads for fear of offending their subscribers with explicit ads. Another controversial aspect is whether such ads encourage and condone sexual activity, especially among teenagers and unmarried people. Various religious groups are particularly upset over this issue and feel the ads encourage sex before marriage and do not encourage abstinence as a means of control.

The other major area for public health efforts is with the community of drug users and abusers. Work needs to be done to prevent and treat drug abuse and to inform the drug abusing community about the dangers of sharing dirty needles. Needles and "works" can be cleaned with bleach if addicts do not have an unlimited supply of clean needles. The issue of distributing free needles to addicts is also a controversial one among health officials, drug enforcement personnel, and local, state, and national government officials.

PSYCHIATRIC INTERVENTIONS

Differential diagnosis to differentiate between organic and functional etiologies. This includes mental status evaluations with particular attention to cognitive functioning. Appropriate work-up may include neurological consultations as well as diagnostic tests such as CAT scan of the head, lumbar puncture, and brain wave testing—EEG.

Not too long ago, when renal transplant patients showed changes in mental status such as alterations in thinking, behavior, and emotion, sepsis was found to be a common cause and astute physicians would first draw a CBC (complete blood count) and start antibiotics. Now, if such a patient has repeated or severe opportunistic infections, one needs to consider HIV infection as another strong possibility. The presence of the AIDS virus will help differentiate an HIV infection in an immunocompromised patient from opportunistic infections secondary to immune suppression alone, such as exists in renal transplant patients (NAPHT 1985).

Treatment of emotional disorders in patients with AIDS and ESRD. The treatment is similar to that of other physically ill patients: helping them deal with their illness by clarifying issues, treatments, and options. Are there any precipitating stresses and if so can they be removed or reduced? If not, can the patient be helped to cope more effectively with them?

In addition there are some issues specific to AIDS and to some of the populations that are afflicted by AIDS. For example, patients may have to deal with revealing their drug addiction or homosexuality for the first time at the same time they are diagnosed as having AIDS. Friends and family may not have known about this aspect of their life.

With respect to counseling and psychotherapy, gay men respond better to personal counseling, either on a one-to-one basis or in groups. The hospice model of dealing with terminally ill patients, as well as modalities that encourage exploration and expression of feelings, can be utilized. Drug addicts, on the other hand, respond poorly to the modalities. They can't sit on or touch feelings; if they could they wouldn't have to inject chemicals and drugs into their bodies. With personal counseling some become worse, act out, and need external controls or they regress. In groups they deny that AIDS exists or that they have it. They project their feelings and beliefs onto society. They need interdisciplinary treatment teams to be effectively treated. If they totally regress they may need psychiatric inpatient hospitalization, especially if they become acutely suicidal and/or psychotic (Bihari 1986).

PHARMACOTHERAPY

There are two main precautions about using psychotropics in renal failure patients. One is that some drugs are dialyzed out and dialysis will reduce their blood levels. These drugs require post dialysis levels for dose adjustment. The second precaution is that drugs that are normally excreted by the kidneys will, if given to patients with renal failure in the same doses as to patients with normal renal function, build up in the body, possibly to toxic proportions.

Psychotropics such as neuroleptics and tricyclic antidepressants are not dialyzable. Benzodiazepines are metabolized by the liver into pharmacologically active metabolites that may accumulate in the presence of renal failure. Therefore it is best to avoid those medications with active metabolites. It is also advisable to use doses that are two-thirds the dose given to regular patients and to monitor dose and response.

Lithium is dialyzable and also excreted by the kidneys. It can be used, however, if certain precautions are observed. After each hemodialysis run, a fixed dose—for example, 600 mg—is given, and since there is no excretion by the kidneys, that amount stays in the body until the next dialysis, when it is removed. When that dialysis run is completed, another dose is administered. Lithium levels are monitored frequently to avoid toxicity (O'Connell, Mahony, and Sheil 1985).

Patients who have behavioral disturbances secondary to deliria and/or dementia such as uremic and/or AIDS encephalopathy may need to be rapidly tranquilized to prevent harm to themselves or others. The drug that I prefer is Haloperidol (Haldol); it can be given orally, intramuscularly or intravenously. A method for treating deliria with intravenous Haldol has been described by Levy (1985). Patients who have irreversible brain damage — dementia, secondary to either the AIDS virus or dialytic dementia — may need maintenance neuroleptics to control disruptive behavior, in addition to placement in supervised settings. Other medications such as antidepressants, lithium carbonate, psychostimulants, and anxiolytics have been used with AIDS patients with varying degrees of success (Adams 1984).

REFERENCES

Adams, F. "Neuropsychiatric Evaluation and Treatment of Delirium in the Critically Ill Cancer Patient." *Cancer Bulletin* 36:156-160.

"AIDS: Deadly But Hard to Catch." 1986, November. *Consumer Reports*, pp. 724-728.

"AIDS and Race." 198, March 10. *Village Voice*, p. 23.

Bihari, B., J. Fine, F. Cancellari, and Z. Mohammed. 1986. "AIDS the Disease and Its Spectre." Paper presented at psychiatric grand rounds, SUNY Health Science Center at Brooklyn, November 15.

Bobbey, P. M. 1987, June 1. *The New York Times*.

Centers for Disease Control. 1986. "Recommendations for Providing Dialysis Treatment to Patients Infected with Human Lymphotropic Virus Type III/Lymphadenopathy-Associated Virus." *MMWR* 35:376-378.

Comomy, J. P. 1982. "Treatment of Certain Metabolic Encephalopathies." In W. C. Weiderholt, ed. *Therapy for Neurologic Disorders*. New York: John Wiley and Sons, pp. 15-23.

"Cost of AIDS Care Is Half What Was Projected, Economist Reports." 1986, June 8. *New York Times*, p. 30.

Cummings, N. B. and S. Klahr. 1985. New York: Plenum Publishing Co.

Delley, J. W., E. E. Shelp, and S. L. Batki. 1986. "Psychiatric and Ethical Issues in the Care of Patients with AIDS." *Psychosomatics* 27:562-566.

Delley, J. W., H. N. Ochitill et al. 1985. "Findings in Psychiatric Consultations with Patients with Acquired Immune Deficiency Syndrome." *American Journal of Psychiatry* 142:82-86.

De-Nour, A. K. 1976. "The Psychiatric Aspects of Renal Hemodialysis." In J. G. Howells, ed. *Modern Perspectives in the Psychiatric Aspects of Surgery*. New York: Brunner/Mazel, pp. 343-375.

Dubovsky, S. L. and I. Penn. 1980. "Psychiatric Considerations in Renal Transplant Surgery." *Psychosomatics* 21:481-490.

Eisendrath, R. M. 1976. "Adaptation to Renal Transplantation." In J. G. Howells, Ed. *Modern Perspectives in the Psychiatric Aspects of Surgery*. New York: Brunner/Mazel, pp. 376-389.

Goldman, M., J. L. Vanherweghem, C. Liesnard et al. 1986. "More on AIDS in Patients on Dialysis" [letter]. *New England Journal of Medicine* 314:1386-1387.

"Inmates Said to Put AIDS Serum in Coffee." 1986, July 26. *New York Times*.

Klein, R. S. 1986. "More on AIDS in Patients on Dialysis" [letter]. *New England Journal of Medicine* 314:1386.

Levy, N. B. 1977. "Psychological Studies at the Downstate Medical Center of Patients on Hemodialysis." *Medical Clinics of North America* 61:759-769.

Levy, N. B. 1979a. "How to Manage and Support Patients on Hemodialysis." *Behavioral Medicine* May:21-24.

Levy, N. B. 1979b. "The Sexual Rehabilitation of the Hemodialysis Patient." *Sexuality and Disability* 2:60-65.

Levy, N. B. 1985. "Use of Psychotropics in Patients with Kidney Failure." *Psychosomatics* 26:699-709.

Margreiter, R., D. Fuchs, A. Hausen et al. 1986. "HIV Infection in Renal Allograft Recipients" [letter]. *Lancet* 2:398.

McKegney, F. P. 1986. AIDS: Fears and Facts. *Psychiatric News* 21 November, pp. 8-9.

National Association of Patients on Hemodialysis and Transplantation. 1986. "NAPHT Drafts AIDS Guidelines for Renal Community." *Dialysis and Transplantation Today*. May, p. 267.

National Institutes of Mental Health. 1986. *Coping with AIDS*. Washington, D.C.: U.S. Government Printing Office.

Neumayer, H., K. Wagner, and S. Kresse. 1986. "HTLV-III Antibodies in Patients with Kidney Transplants or on Haemodialysis" [letter]. *Lancet* 1:497.

Nichols, S. E. 1985. "Psychosocial Reactions of Persons with the Acquired Immunodeficiency Syndrome." *Annals of Internal Medicine* 103:765-767.

O'Connell, P. J., J. F. Mahony, and A. G. R. Sheil. "AIDS After Renal Transplantation: [letter]. *The Medical Journal of Australia* 143:631.

"Psychological Sequelae May Be Signs of AIDS." 1985. *Clinical Psychiatry News* 13(10):12.

Rao, T. K. S., E. J. Filippone, A. D. Nicastri et al. 1984. "Associated Focal and Segmental Glomerulosclerosis in the Acquired Immunodeficiency Syndrome." *New England Journal of Medicine* 310:669-673.

Rao, T. K. S., E. A. Friedman, and A. D. Nicastry. "The Types of Renal Disease in the Acquired Immunodeficiency Syndrome." *New England Journal of Medicine* 316:1062-1068.

Steinberg, J. and N. B. Levy. 1979. "Psychiatric Factors in Renal Transplantation." In S. N. Chatterjee, ed. *Manual of Renal Transplantation*. New York: Springer-Verlag, pp. 167-173.

Stewart, R. S. 1984. "The Renal Transplant/Dialysis Unit." In F. G. Guggenheim and M. F. Weiner, eds. *Manual of Psychiatric Consultation and Emergency Care*. New York: Jason Aronson, pp. 307-315.

Sullivan, R. 1987. May 1. *The New York Times*.

"Synthesized Drug Eases Kidney Ills." 1986, January 1. *The New York Times*.

United States Public Health Service and World Health Organization. 1987. Third International Conference on AIDS. Washington, D.C., June 1-5.

Wellisch, D. K. 1985. "UCLA Psychological Study of AIDS." *Frontiers of Radiation Therapy in Oncology* 18:155-158.

"Who Pays for AIDS." 1986. *Nature* 327:548.

Psychosocial Issues in AIDS/ESRD

Thelma Myers

End-stage renal disease (ESRD) is frequently associated with psychosocial problems. Psychosocial difficulties related to a number of causes are seen in patients with ESRD, including depression, dependency on a machine for survival, presence of a chronic illness, alteration of body image, and alteration of role in family relationships. A patient with acquired immune deficiency syndrome (AIDS) also has many of these same psychosocial problems because of the nature of the disease. When a patient with AIDS also has ESRD, many of these problems are compounded, and will require special attention by health care providers to meet the needs of the patient. A number of nursing diagnoses can be identified that would apply to the patient with ESRD and AIDS. Some of the primary problems will be identified with characteristics that caregivers may see, followed by interventions that may help to alleviate the problem.

Anxiety related to the nature of the disease, fear of the unknown, and uncertainty about the future are problems common to both AIDS and ESRD. Anxiety may range from mild to severe. Mild anxiety may be manifested by questioning, restlessness, and increased awareness. Moderate anxiety may be manifested by voice tremors, shakiness, increased muscle tension, increased heart rate, and increased verbalization. Severe anxiety may be manifested by inappropriate verbalization, loss of perceptual focus, tachycardia, and hyperventilation. Health care providers can help to decrease a person's anxiety by offering explanations of all procedures and treatments that are being done, allowing the patient to ask ques-

---

Thelma Myers, RN, is affiliated with the Department of Education, Research and Development, The Presbyterian Hospital in the City of New York, NY.

tions, even when the same questions have been answered before. If an underlying cause of the anxiety can be identified, such as an alteration in comfort, that problem should be addressed and solved to assist in alleviating the anxiety. For example, if a patient is having pain, as is common in patients requiring dialysis and patients with AIDS, relieving the pain will help to decrease anxiety and also help to establish a sense of trust in the caregiver. A number of resources are available to the hospitalized patient, and they should be utilized to help decrease anxiety. Some of these resources include social services, chaplains, other patients with the same problems, and psychiatrists. When simple measures do not help to decrease a person's anxiety, it will be necessary to utilize other resources. If necessary, medications may be used to help control anxiety, at least initially.

Depression is another problem that is seen in patients with AIDS and patients with ESRD. The literature documents that any chronic disease may cause depression in many patients. The chronicity of the disease and the need for continued treatment causes patients to experience a feeling of helplessness leading to depression. ESRD requiring lifelong dialysis that disrupts a person's normal routines of life is distressing to many people. In a person with ESRD and AIDS, that depression may be even greater. In addition to having a disease that requires chronic treatment to stay alive, that person has a diagnosis of a disease that is almost universally fatal. The helplessness and hopelessness associated with a fatal disease complicates the need for a chronic treatment to sustain life. Patients often question the rationale to continue a complicated treatment program when the ultimate outcome of their disease is almost certain death. Dealing with these feelings in the patient with AIDS and ESRD is also difficult for health care providers. Often patients with AIDS are young adults with their whole lives ahead of them. A disease without a treatment is so uncommon in our society that health care providers also react with feelings of helplessness and hopelessness. Addressing these needs of the patient with AIDS requires all the resources that a facility can provide. Psychiatric evaluation may be necessary to identify the most effective approach to dealing with the depression that accompanies a patient's physical problems.

Social isolation is a problem that many patients with ESRD have identified. Patients who require dialysis treatments three times a week and who have to follow a strict diet and fluid restriction have frequently complained that they feel isolated from their family and friends. Patients with AIDS suffer even more from these feelings of isolation. Often, their families and friends are not available to offer the support they need. Because of our society's prejudices, many patients with AIDS have suffered societal rejection. Because a large number of patients with AIDs are either intravenous drug abusers or homosexual or bisexual men, our society's prejudices against these groups have extended to patients with AIDS. The high risk groups associated with AIDS evoke many feelings and attitudes in our society; these attitudes are also found among health care workers. Groups that are different from what we consider "the norm" are seen as socially unacceptable and receive the brunt of our prejudices. A common reaction is withdrawal and avoidance of these people. When confronted with the knowledge of a chronic and fatal disease, these patients require all the support and understanding they can get. What they do not need is for family, friends, and health care providers to avoid them. One possible solution to the problem of social isolation is to help educate family and friends. Many people are not aware of the modes of transmission and may be afraid of acquiring the disease from casual association with the patient. Family and friends can be assured that transmission of the disease occurs through sexual contact and through blood-to-blood contact. Misconceptions about high risk groups can also be dispelled. Many people have preconceived ideas about homosexuals and intravenous drug abusers that are not accurate. For example, one common myth about intravenous drug abusers is that they are all street people and live in shelters. In actuality, IVDA crosses all ages, races, and social levels. The IVDA may be a Wall Street executive or a physician or the man living in the shelter. Stereotypic ideas about male homosexuals are just as erroneous, but just as prevalent in our society. Helping family, friends, and health care workers to recognize their misconceptions can also help to provide better care to the patient. Involving family or friends in the care of patients can help greatly to eliminate the feelings of isolation and loneliness. Patients with chronic diseases have a great need to know that they are accepted and loved; nurses can help to provide this support. If no family members are available, providing the patient with other contacts — social services, volunteers, chaplains, and outside organizations such as Gay Men's Health Crisis — is very important.

Another commonly seen problem is alteration in self-image. Patients on dialysis have frequently complained of an alteration in their self-image because of vascular access, weight loss or gain, and changes in physical stamina. These are also problems in patients with AIDS. A change in appearance as well as a change in physical abilities is frequently seen in patients with AIDS. In patients with AIDS, physical changes may occur because of skin lesions or weight loss. Other changes in self-image occur because of an inability to function at previous levels of activity. Fatigue and malaise are frequently complaints of patients with ESRD as well as patients with AIDS. Even before a patient has a definite diagnosis of AIDS, he or she may have gone through a period of decreasing physical stamina that affected his or her usual lifestyle. Many patients will not be able to continue to function at their usual jobs or fulfill their family responsibilities. Decreased levels of activity can contribute to and cause many other social problems. If the person is unable to maintain his or her job, financial needs will develop requiring even more social assistance. In dealing with the problem of decreased self-image, health care workers can encourage patients to continue as many activities as they are able and to provide assistance to maintain the maximum level of function. Patients can also be assured of their acceptance despite possible physical changes in appearance or changes in level of activity.

Going along with changes in self-image, alteration in self-care activities is frequently seen. Patients with ESRD frequently experience decreased ability to perform their usual routines. Patients with AIDS also experience these problems. Chronic fatigue from ESRD or AIDS can require a total change in a person's usual level of activities. A formerly athletic person may have difficulty even performing usual activities of daily living. If the necessary assistance (physical as well as emotional) is not available, many other problems can evolve from this inability to perform self-care activities. For example, if a patient with AIDS is too tired to prepare his food, his nutritional intake is not going to be adequate and will predispose him to other physical problems. If nutrition is inadequate, the person is more susceptible to infections, skin breakdown, and further decrease in tolerance to activity. Social resources in the community are limited, but should be identified to assist the patient to maintain as much self-care as possible. Maintaining as much activity as possible will help to maintain a feeling of self-control, will improve self-image, and will help to provide a feeling of hope and worth in the person. Allowing the person as much independence as possible should be encouraged. At the same time, when the person's physical needs warrant it, help needs to be provided so that further problems and complications do not occur.

Any patient with ESRD may have many psychosocial problems or needs in various stages of his disease. Likewise, any patient with a diagnosis of AIDS is likely to also have many psychosocial problems. When a patient with ESRD has AIDS, the psychosocial needs may be even greater and will require a concerted effort by all health care providers to meet these needs. As health care workers, we all need to increase our awareness of these problems and develop a plan to meet these needs.

Psychosocial Factors in the Care of the Geriatric Nephrology Patient

Neima Itschaki

In the early days of dialysis, when health care resources were scarce and funding limited, patients 45 years of age or older were seldom considered for chronic dialysis programs. However, as increased state and federal funding, particularly Medicare, became available, virtually all patients with end-stage renal disease (ESRD) became eligible for treatment—including a significant number of elderly individuals. These people present unique problems for the caretakers.

The purpose of this paper is to review the psychosocial issues inherent in aging, with special attention to the psychosocial needs of the elderly with ESRD.

Old age is a unique experience that depends on an intricate balance of physical, emotional, and social factors in one's life. In old age, deficits in one or several of these areas are common and result in great discomfort to the individual.

Adaptation to the demands of life calls for learning and developing new modes of behavior relevant to the various stages of life. Havighurst (1953) suggests six developmental tasks of later maturity: (1) adjusting to decreasing physical strength and health; (2) adjusting to retirement and reduced income; (3) adjusting to the death of a spouse; (4) establishing an explicit affiliation with one's age group; (5) meeting social and civic obligations; and (6) establishing satisfactory living arrangements. Louis Lowy (1963) identifies four problem areas: (1) gradual isolation and aloneness; (2) the loss of

Neima Itschaki, MS, CSW, is Senior Social Worker and Supervisor, Department of Social Work, Lenox Hill Hospital, New York, NY.

211

social identity; (3) physical and mental loss; and (4) lack of future and fear of death.

BACKGROUND INFORMATION ON THE ELDERLY

In the twentieth century, a phenomenal growth in the population of older individuals has occurred, both in numbers and in their proportion relative to other age groups. From 1900 to 1970, the 60 plus age group grew from 6.4 percent to 14.8 percent of the population. At the same time, fertility of the younger cohorts dropped, which implies fewer children to share the burden of care for the elderly (Bengtson and Treas 1980). Furthermore, with the presently declining birth rate, medical advances, and improved health care delivery, it is anticipated that the percentage of elderly in our population will continue to grow. Of our elderly population, women significantly outnumber men, and proportionally whites outnumber blacks. In regard to marital status, most elderly men are married, while most elderly women are widows. In fact, two-thirds of all older women are widows. Approximately two out of every ten older people in the United States live alone. The loneliest and most isolated people appear to be those widowed persons who have no children and live alone. Social isolation and isolation due to perceptual losses can have profound debilitating effects on the elderly. A serious illness can devastate a person who is alone, since there is no one to care for him or her (Butler and Lewis 1973).

Five percent of the elderly live in institutions while 95 percent still live in the community. Approximately 70 percent of the elderly live in families, i.e., with a spouse, children, or friends, and 25 percent live alone. The elderly live most frequently in central parts of cities or in rural locations, with between 30 and 40 percent of the elderly living in substandard housing (Butler and Lewis 1973).

In regard to income, at retirement, income usually drops 50 percent or more, and during the years that follow, it deteriorates even further. Fifty-two percent of the elderly's income comes from retirement and welfare programs, and the remainder from investment and contributions from relatives. Many elderly continue to work past age 65, and for many, income from work constitutes about 31 percent of their aggregate income (Butler 1975). Yet, as much as half of the elderly in the United States may live in poverty and deprivation, lacking food, essential drugs, adequate housing, and so on. The elderly are the fastest growing poverty group in society. Widows, single women, and members of minority groups are particularly disadvantaged economically (Butler 1975, Butler and Lewis 1973).

The physical health of the majority of the elderly is better than is generally believed. Eighty-one percent of those 65 years and over are fully ambulatory and independent. Nevertheless, old people experience a good deal more acute and chronic diseases than the younger population. Perceptual losses of eyesight and hearing can deplete energy and cause social isolation (Butler and Lewis 1973). The elderly account for 25 percent of the nation's health expenditures because of their great need for medical services and their costlier illnesses. Older people require more physician time and more frequent and longer hospital admissions (Butler 1975).

In addition, anxiety, much of which is rooted in the generalized fear of growing old and becoming dependent, often becomes chronic in old age. And indeed, the mental health needs of the elderly are substantial. Emotional and mental illnesses escalate over the course of the life cycle. Depression, in particular, rises with age, and suicide reaches peak rates in white men in their eighties. The elderly account for approximately 25 percent of the nation's suicide rate (Manney 1975). Depression and hypochondria commonly accompany the many physical diseases of old age. Fear and anxiety grow real with illness. Often the close association between mental and physical health is ignored by health care professionals.

As to family relations, contrary to the common belief, most children continue to care for their parents until they die. Adult children and their elderly parents maintain very strong emotional ties, ongoing contacts, shared social activities, and exchange of material and nonmaterial aid. Family relations contribute to the mental health and sense of well-being of the elderly (Bengtson and Treas 1980). Families that do not offer help to their older members do so because of a variety of personal, financial, and social reasons rather than an attitude of neglect (Birren 1964, Butler and Lewis 1973).

Older persons experience more stresses than any other age group, at a time of already depleted resources for coping with these stresses. Change, loss, and grief are the predominant themes characterizing the emotional experiences of old age (Butler 1975). Losses in every aspect of late life force the elderly to expend enormous amounts of physical and emotional energy in mourning and resolving grief, adapting to the changes that result from loss, and recovering from the stresses inherent in these processes. As Butler and Lewis (1973) describe,

> The elderly are confronted by multiple losses, which may occur simultaneously: death of a marital partner, older friends, colleagues, relatives; decline of physical health and coming to personal terms with death; loss of status, prestige and participation in society; and for large numbers of the older population, additional burdens of marginal living standards. (p. 29)

Depression, anxiety, psychosomatic illnesses, paranoia, and irritability are some of the reactions to these stresses (Butler 1975).

THE ELDERLY PATIENT WITH ESRD

In an earlier publication this author, together with Dr. Joel Gonchar, presented an extensive discussion on the psychosocial factors in the care of the geriatric nephrology patient:

> These people present unique problems. Stresses of growing old, discussed earlier, are compounded by the devastating effects of a chronic disease that imposes severe limitations on the functioning and the lifestyle of the elderly. Confinement to the dialysis machine, time commitment, loss of freedom, and the demand for rigid compliance to diet and fluid restrictions, require major alterations of lifestyle. Most patients are dialyzed 2-3 times a week for 4-5 hours each time. Important life events, such as recreation, social and family life, traveling, and, often, even work, become secondary in importance to this life-sustaining therapy. Freedom of movement is limited, ironically, at this stage of life when the patient is no longer tied to work and to child-rearing responsibilities. Most elderly peo-

ple look forward to retirement as a time to fulfill desires, dreams, and hopes of various kinds before they die. The prospect of being tied to a treatment and the strict lifestyle demanded by dialysis becomes particularly discouraging from this point of view. Many elderly patients become bitter and express feelings of being cheated in life.

As stated earlier, adjustment to changes in life deploys all biological, psychological, and social resources available to the individual. Keeping in mind that old age is a time when many losses are experienced, the loss of kidney function adds to the depletion of these resources. Mourning for the loss of body function, shock, depression, anger, and despair, are some of the common emotional reactions expressed by many elderly patients with ESRD. Further, many experience frustration and a deep sense of deprivation due to an inability to engage in enjoyable activities that require physical stamina. Most experience an increased sense of fragility and a deep anxiety about further deterioration in their health and increased need for dependency on others—a concern of great magnitude for those who live alone. However, when other body systems are still intact, many elderly ESRD patients are able to enjoy a fruitful and active life for quite a number of years. In many of these cases, the ability to restore a normal life depends very much on the patient's emotional strength and the availability of a supportive family and social network. Other elderly ESRD patients who present with multisystem diseases or several illnesses at the same time, become devastatingly depleted, especially if these conditions linger over a long period of time. Emotional and financial resources of family members are also depleted as they struggle to cope with the stresses of the patient's illness. Issues of quality of life may be raised by both the patient, the family, and staff members, who may feel discouraged by their inability to help the patient. A few patients may opt to terminate dialysis in the absence of meaningful and pleasurable experiences in their lives.

Patients with ESRD do not get better. They will be on dialysis therapy for the rest of their lives. Dependency on medical staff is greater for dialysis patients than with any other disease due to the frequency of treatment (Gonchar and Itschaki 1986, p. 155).

In a study conducted by McKevitt and Kappel (1977) on 24 chronic patients 58 years of age and older, the authors found that these people's concerns were basically focused on health, maintaining independence, finances, and securing medical care. Other major sources of concern for the elderly on dialysis are lack of energy, health problems of self and family members, and concerns about ability to care for self in the future. Another issue that these patients related was loneliness. Although most of them maintain close contacts with family and friends, almost 60 percent of them reported feeling lonely at least some of the time. Depression was also prevalent among these people. One-third of the patients felt at times that life wasn't worth living, and one-fourth of the patients have at times considered discontinuing treatment. Other significant sources of concern were income, sexual functioning, finding help in an emergency, and provision of drugs and transportation to dialysis.

SERVICES TO THE ELDERLY WITH ESRD

Elderly patients with ESRD require a whole range of services that involve the complete cooperation of various incenter disciplines, such as medicine, nursing, social work, nutrition, and psychiatry, and a variety of community services. The patients and their families require continuous advice and interpretation of the medical, technical, and dietary aspects of their care. They need a great deal of support and encouragement from all staff members and psychosocial counseling to help them cope with the stresses of their illness. Many need special home care services, especially if they live alone or with an infirm spouse. Some require ambulette transportation to and from dialysis. Only a few require institutionalization. All these services are costly, and, when provided over a long period of time, deplete the family's financial resources and become a source of concern to both the patient and the surviving spouse.

When such services are provided by government programs, they can be fragmented, limited, and they may require a long wait. The health care team is especially necessary at such times for helping the patient and his family acquire and utilize available resources (Gonchar and Itschaki 1986, pp. 157-158).

Social work counseling and the intervention of other team members must acknowledge the importance of patients' concerns and fears about loss of control, loneliness, depression, and sexual functioning. Assisting and encouraging the patients to become knowledgeable about, and active participants in, their own care will help them gain a sense of involvement, control, and mastery in their treatment situation. Patients should also be encouraged to express their loneliness and need for support and companionship. Barriers or problems influencing the quality of relationships should be explored, while engaging the patients and their family members in an active process of enriching these relationships. Patients should also be encouraged to expand their support systems by increasing participation in church groups and community or volunteer activities. Social workers, in collaboration with other team members, can help the patients ventilate their feelings of loss, discouragement, and depression. McKevitt and Kappel (1977) state,

> We should explore with and elicit from patients, methods, techniques, or problem-solving approaches which may help them to deal with and obtain some relief from the discomfort of depressed feelings (p. 48).

If depression appears severe, consultation and/or intervention by a psychiatrist may be necessary.

SUMMARY

A chronic disease such as ESRD compounds the stresses of growing old, imposes severe limitations on the physical and psychosocial functioning of the elderly, and is a major source of stress for the family. Intense staff involvement with the patient and his or her family are necessary in the form of emotional support, encouragement, advice, emotional counseling, and arrangements for necessary supportive social and home services.

REFERENCES

Bengtson, V. L. and J. Treas. 1980. "The Changing Family Context of Mental Health and Aging." In J. Birren and B. Sleave, eds. *Handbook of Mental Health and Aging*. Englewood Cliffs, NJ: Prentice-Hall, Inc.

Birren, J. 1964. *The Psychology of Aging*. Englewood Cliffs, NJ: Prentice-Hall, Inc.

Butler, R. N. 1975. *Why Survive? Being Old in America*. New York: Harper and Row.

Butler, R. N. and M. L. Lewis. 1973. *Aging and Mental Health: Positive Psychological Approaches*. St. Louis, MO: C. V. Mosby Co.

Gonchar, J. and N. Itschaki. 1986. "Psychosocial Factors in the Geriatric Nephrology Patient." In M. F. Michelis, B. B. Davis, and H. G. Preuss, eds. *Geriatric Nephrology*. New York: Field, Rich and Associates, Inc.

Havighurst, R. J. 1953. *Human Development and Education*. New York: David McKay Co.

Lowy, L. 1963. "Meeting the Needs of Older People on a Differential Basis." In *Social Group Work with Older People*. New York: National Association of Social Workers.

Manney, J. D. Jr. 1975. *Aging in American Society: An Examination of Concepts and Issues*. Ann Arbor, MI: Wayne State University Institute of Gerontology.

McKevitt, P. and D. Kappel. 1977. "Psychosocial Needs and Concerns of the Elderly on Dialysis." *Perspectives: The Journal of the Council on Nephrology Social Workers* 2(1).

T - #0244 - 101024 - C0 - 212/152/12 [14] - CB - 9781560241492 - Gloss Lamination